SUCCESSFUL AGING

OTHER BOOKS BY OLGA KNOPF
The Art of Being a Woman
Women on Their Own

Successful Aging

OLGA KNOPF, M.D.

*With the editorial assistance
of Phyllis Freeman*

THE VIKING PRESS

New York

To the memory of Erni

LIBRARY OF CONGRESS CATALOGING IN PUBLICATION DATA

Knopf, Olga, 1888-
  Successful aging.

  Bibliography: p.
  1. Aged—United States. 2. Old age. 3. Aging.
I. Title.
HQ1064.U5K5   1975   301.43'4   74-19250
ISBN 0-670-68081-8

Printed in U.S.A.

Contents

. . . growing old, it's not nice,

but it's interesting.

—AUGUST STRINDBERG

Acknowledgments

*I*t is almost harder to enumerate the many people to whom I am indebted for assistance in this study—especially those whose publications enlarged my knowledge and stimulated my thinking—than it was to do the writing itself. As the reader can see, this study is the result of more than thirty years of interest, observation, reading, and talking to people. It was therefore impossible to list all my sources. Instead, I have confined myself to naming in the text only the authors whom I have drawn on directly. May the many more from whom I learned and to whom I want to express gratitude at this time forgive me if I have omitted them.

There are, however, a few people to whom I owe specific gratitude—most of all, my friend of forty years, Miriam Wolf, who was godmother to the book. It was she with whom I discussed many ideas as they germinated in my mind, and it was her understanding and encouragement that kept me writing in the beginning when the going was rough.

I want to express my special appreciation to Dr. Alvin I. Goldfarb, associate clinical professor of psychiatry, Mount Sinai School of Medicine, for generously sharing his broad knowledge of the treatment and management of the mentally disturbed aged. His many publications on this and related subjects helped me a great deal in formulating my own views about the kind of aged with whom I am communicating here.

I am most grateful to Dr. Lawrence J. Roose, Clinical Professor of Psychiatry, Mount Sinai School of Medicine, for making it possible for me to visit with the aged patients on some medical wards, where I had the opportunity to observe the ways they faced the terminal portions of their lives.

Special thanks are due to Barbara Burn, my editor at Viking, who responded to my telephone call offering the book that had not yet been completed. It was her confidence in my ability to present this subject competently that sustained my courage while I was working. I also owe a debt of gratitude to Phyllis Freeman, who, although young in years, showed remarkable ability to identify with my subject and to assist me in expressing my thoughts appropriately.

My thanks are extended also to my personal friends, whom I bored with my preoccupation with my subject, and to my friends and colleagues in the hospital, who checked up regularly on the progress of my writing.

Introduction

HOW THIS BOOK CAME TO BE WRITTEN

*T*hroughout the course of human evolution, the aged have always held a precarious place in the group to which they have belonged. When the group was threatened in its existence by a famine, the weaker members—the sick and the infirm aged—were the first ones to be sacrificed in favor of the survival of the stronger ones. If the tribe had to flee from an attacker, the less mobile members—again the sick and the infirm aged—were abandoned on the flight.

As societies became less nomadic and settled in a fixed location, the need to live together with the smallest risk to the safety of the individual members led to the formulation of moral codes. In the early days of our civilization, the Ten Commandments appeared—living proof of these ancient attempts to harness human tendencies that, if left unbridled, would endanger the existence of the group as a whole. No commandments would have been necessary unless the group had had to curb temptation for the sake of the common good.

One of the commandments most often cited is: "Honor thy Father and thy Mother." Civilization has reached increasingly higher levels, but the observance of that commandment seems not to have kept pace. Granted that the aged and the infirm are no longer left by the wayside to shift for themselves and to die of hunger in solitude; granted that most families live on good terms with their aged members. Nevertheless, the old as a group have by no means been "honored" by society. It is almost astonishing that nations today, with their solicitude for the destinies of remote peoples, should have to be awakened to the fact that a large number of their own old people live on a substandard level of existence, lonely and all but forgotten by the rest of the population. Old people without families, or those whose state of health was such that they could no longer be kept at home, have never been very popular. In earlier days—and until a few years ago in parts of the United States—it was standard practice to shove them into poorhouses; if the community lacked even this facility, they were put in a jail or insane asylum, where they ended their days in misery. Because they had no ways of controlling or even complaining about their fate, their cases seldom came to public attention.

It was not until the mid-1930s, with the introduction of Social Security, that the first large-scale meaningful steps were taken to make life more bearable for the aged. The concept of the Social Security laws was, in my belief, a stroke of genius. Coming at the depth of the Depression, when jobs were hard to get, it changed the working and living patterns of virtually the entire population. By instituting the possibility of retirement at sixty-five, coupled with the simultaneous extension of compulsory schooling from fourteen to sixteen years, the government reduced the labor supply and eliminated the two groups who could afford, and were often compelled, to work for the lowest wages: the very young and the very old. This contraction in the number of job-seekers gave mature men and women who were still responsible for rearing a family a better chance of having a job, and at something like decent wages. In addition, old people were protected from total want by Social Security payments, certainly modest at that time, but a protection just the same.

No matter how inspired and necessary this measure was, and no matter how beneficial for the majority of wage earners, it, like many other laws supposedly designed to help the older generation, proved a mixed blessing: though many now received a pension, a large number of aging people who were healthy and able to work were suddenly eliminated from the labor market and put on short rations.

The psychological impact this nationwide occurrence had on the family and on the role of the aged in society became clear in the short span of ten years. In the mid-1940s, a group of high-school students were asked whether they felt they should be responsible for the support of their parents in old age; more than half said no. To a middle-aged person, such as I was at that time, this was simple heresy. What was more, many young workers resented the deductions from their paychecks for their own future Social Security, saying it was their money that supported the current recipients. Some remnants of this misconception persist to this day; they do not enhance the popularity of the aged in general.

Another very important consequence of compulsory retirement was that until this practice was introduced, age as such did not enter into the evaluation of a person, especially a worker, nor did it alter his social position so long as he was able to pull his weight. In primitive as well as early societies, we find numerous examples of the high esteem aged men and women enjoyed. One cannot help admiring the resourcefulness with which they held on to this preferential treatment within their group in spite of the lessening of their physical vigor—a characteristic of major importance in nomadic societies. The elders of the group, the heroes and warriors who survived, became the advisers in the tribe's policies. They negotiated war and peace with other groups, became judges and arbiters among their own members; they were priests, which meant that they were the intermediaries between the living and the spirits; they knew how to pacify the hostile deities and how to reward the friendly ones. As Leo W. Simmons reported in his excellent study,* it was the elders who decided which parts of a sacrificed animal were taboo for mortals and had to be left for the spirits. Simmons must have had a twinkle in his eye when he remarked on the toothlessness of the aged priests, who, after the sacrificial feast, helped themselves to the soft parts, which they had declared taboo. Their ingenuity makes one glad they succeeded.

The old were also held in esteem as the historians in any society that had not yet developed writing; the history of the tribe, the customs, the traditions, the records of their heroic deeds were transmitted from one generation to the next by word of mouth. They also were the medicine men and women, who knew the herbs that healed and those that poisoned; they could foretell the future and exert their influence with the spirits to make rain or stop it. It took a long time to acquire all this knowledge, and very few of the group lived long enough to master these complicated rituals. However, as soon as one of these old people fell into dotage, he was no longer held in awe. From then on, he was neither useful nor a threat to anyone, and in time of stress he was abandoned with the rest of the sick to shift for himself.

As private property developed, the old people of these periods were just as much catered to as are those who hold the purse strings today. They, too, fell from grace once they reached dotage.

The power of the purse has clouded the real role of the aged in later societies. In the recent past, the "man of the house" seems to have enjoyed more status than he does now—because he was the sole wage earner in the family. His wife exerted a great deal of influence over the children—because she was the dispenser of the

* *The Role of the Aged in Primitive Society* (New Haven: Yale University Press, 1945).

family income. And the earnings of the children—as long as they lived at home—also belonged to the parents. All these facts do not testify to the love and esteem a parent received in old age from his children. But the family structure was different until the turn of this century, and the position of aged parents was generally less precarious.

It was left to the era of Social Security and compulsory retirement to make men and women age-conscious. Since the first days of Social Security, much progress has been made, but it has not been quick enough or far-reaching enough to afford lasting and adequate relief. A number of fervent and articulate champions of the cause of the aged have made themselves heard, but in their eagerness to draw attention to the acute need of old people, they have overstressed the negative aspects of old age and underestimated the potential of old people. In defense of these voices "in the wilderness," one rather important factor must be taken into consideration: anyone who champions a cause fights at the same time a private battle within himself. A writer or a scientist who becomes interested enough in any aspect of life to make a systematic study of it has usually been struggling with the same problem in his own life or within his family. Doing research and finally writing about it represent an attempt to come to grips with a personal cause. Therefore, an author cannot be expected to be completely objective in dealing with his subject. I am no exception.

For personal reasons, when I was in my middle fifties, more than twenty-five years ago, I became interested in the relationship between middle-aged adults and their aged parents. I tried to follow the old rule that one learns best by teaching: I had been giving courses on psychological subjects at the New School for Social Research in New York City for eighteen years. I devoted the next two years to lecturing specifically on the topic of adults and their parents. Subsequently, I accepted a contract to write a book on this subject. I did a great deal of research, held numerous interviews with families, talked with friends and patients. Up to that time, I had thought of myself as being broad-minded and tolerant of other people, but to my great dismay, I was not able to attain the necessary objectivity in my evaluation of the sources of conflict between the generations. In spite of my experience as a psychiatrist, I found myself prejudiced against the aged, so much so that I reluctantly came to the conclusion that my bias would prevent me from doing justice to the topic. I solved my dilemma at that time by returning the contract; the book remained unwritten.

My awareness of this prejudice and its background never left me, and neither did the guilt feeling about my attitude. As time went on, I realized that I was not the only one who felt this way; I could see how deeply this prejudice against the aged had pervaded our society. Digging further into the problem, and studying the results of research by experts in this field, I began to understand that there were certain unconscious mechanisms causing this almost universal rejection of the aged.

By the time I had progressed in my understanding of both generations—the aged and the near-aged—I had passed through both stages and become aged myself. I knew the whole process from personal experience.

When I became seventy-three, I found that I was no longer strong enough to carry the sole responsibility for a number of sick people. In preparation for retirement, I started to reduce the number of hours I spent with patients by not accepting new ones. Since I began to have time on my hands, I experimented with various leisure activities. I finally ended up with a busman's holiday— conducting a discussion group on topics of interest to members of a large day-care center for older people. I also saw quite a few of the members in individual consultation and thus learned a great deal about old people other than myself.

After two years, I gave up this volunteer activity, and in the spring of 1965, I was invited to join the staff of the Institute of Psychiatry at Mount Sinai Hospital in New York City. My function was to be a preceptor (supervisor and instructor) in geriatrics at the institute, as part of its training program. Staff members had observed that some of the aged patients were reluctant to talk to the young residents, and they felt that these patients might prefer to talk to a contemporary, and therefore profit more from their stay at the hospital. This is how I received my appointment—because of my age rather than in spite of it—and when the new medical school opened, I was also appointed a member of the faculty. I still hold both appointments with great pride and satisfaction.

I had never done this kind of work before, and the challenge was extremely stimulating. My second career was well under way.

After a while, my work with the residents was no longer confined to their aged patients but was extended to include all adult age groups.

Although every patient received expert care from the medical and nursing staff, I noticed, as time went on, that there was a difference in the attitude of the staff toward their young and their old patients. There was a shyness and a reticence on the part of a young resident when he had to take an old person's history, almost like that of a child asking intimate questions of his parent. There was a hesitation on the part of the nursing staff to tell an aged patient what he had to do and to keep him in line—an essential professional function, since every patient has to adjust to the patient community. Several of the nursing staff had become aware of these facts themselves but were not able to understand the reasons for them. These barriers left the staff frustrated and the elderly angry because they felt that they were not getting sufficient attention. As a result, these patients felt even more unwanted than when they had been living on the outside.

There was no ill will on either side, just inexperience, which in these cases was owing to lack of knowledge of what it is to be old, what goes on in an old person who lives among young people, what an old one had to put up with before he or she became sick, and what kind of life he will have to return to after his discharge.

All these impressions became intensified when I was assigned the additional task of visiting regularly with the aged patients in some medical wards. These wards were crowded, the staff was overworked, and very little attention could be paid to any aspect aside from the patients' physical condition. Some were admitted to the hospital with terminal diseases in their last stages and actually died a short time after admission. Most of them did not know that their end was near, although they may have felt it; some of them did not want to know; a few were ready to accept the fact that their time was coming to an end.

Much too little is known about this phase of human life, about the world the aged live in; what the interaction is between their inner life and their physical and economic situation. Still less is known about the interrelationship between the old one and his family and society at large, especially the rejection—if not ostracism—that he experiences once he is retired and no longer has any voice in the course of events around him. The result of these circumstances is a general pessimism among the aged: a loss of self-respect, a feeling of being a burden to their families and to themselves.

My personal experiences as I became older and finally old, and my dealings with the young and middle-aged generations, renewed my desire to clarify my views to myself and to share them with my contemporaries. Government statisticians group the people from fifty-five to seventy-five and over by ten-year intervals. The middle group (sixty-five to seventy-four) is officially termed the aged; those seventy-five and over are called overaged. And I like to call the first group, from fifty-five to sixty-four, the near-aged.

There are numerous publications about the aged, many statistics about their lives, and a great deal of data about their physical and mental reactions. Yet very few attempts have been made to communicate with the aged. I believe the time has come to talk *to* the aged instead of *about* them.

The aged I am talking to are those who are in fairly good health and still functioning in life. For this reason, I have not included any discussions or explanations of physical and mental conditions caused by illness or by marked deterioration due to advanced aging. By acquainting this group of aged with themselves and explaining the background of the changes in their bodies inherent in the process of aging, and by pointing out the adaptations they must make in their mode of living because of age and retirement, I hope to increase their self-awareness and thus to cushion the sting of the hurt their new role has caused them and to induce them to accept situations they cannot change.

All this necessitates the use of everyday language and the avoidance of technical terms as much as possible. After all, the majority of the present-day aged did not have the opportunity for higher education or any time later on to catch up with the newest discoveries in the sciences. Some of my critics may raise their eyebrows about this lack of technical language and accuse me of superficiality. After twenty years of experience in adult education, I arrived by trial and error at the conclusion that if a person must ponder the meaning of a word too often while reading or studying, he loses the thread of continuity and soon his interest in the subject disappears entirely.

I am at the same time making myself the spokesman for the old generation by explaining to the younger generations the various manifestations of aging—in the hope that I can help the young to bridge the gap between themselves and their elders and simultaneously ease their approach toward their own inescapable future.

The reasons for the almost universal rejection of the aged by the younger generation will also be investigated, and I hope that new insight on both sides will improve the relationship between them by making them more tolerant of each other, for to live in peace with one's family is one of the most important factors in the last stages of our lives.

I will try to show how to organize the daily routine after retirement, how to watch out for pitfalls in our daily lives and avoid unnecessary mishaps and accidents, and what to do when infirmity begins to assert itself.

There have been a great many improvements in the lives of the aged and progress is still being made, but many more objectives await realization. These too will be discussed and ways shown in which we the old can play an active part in bringing these changes about.

Appendix A is devoted to a survey of the extensive facilities available to the aged, which can enable them to take care of their health and organize their lives in the way they want to, according to their own individual means, likes, and dislikes, rather than according to the preconceived ideas of the planners. I myself was surprised to discover the multitude of programs initiated and operated by the federal government on behalf of all groups of our population, including the aged. It is regrettable that so little is known about their existence.

In spite of my diligent research and many years of sustaining the courage of people during their dark hours, I might still not have written this book had it not been for the encouragement and support I received from the staff of the Institute of Psychiatry of the Mount Sinai School of Medicine, beginning with Dr. M. Ralph Kaufman, Esther and Joseph Klingenstein Professor of Psychiatry Emeritus, who gave me the opportunity to work there, and after his retirement, from Dr. Marvin Stein, present holder of this chair and Chairman of the Department of Psychiatry; from my colleagues, all of them many years younger than I; and the residents, who came as fledglings and left as experts. I owe special appreciation to my immediate superior for the first seven years, Dr. Edward D. Joseph, professor of psychiatry at Mount Sinai School of Medicine. Without his consent and encouragement, it would not have been possible to lower from sixty to eighteen the age span of the patients whose treatment by the residents I supervise. Because I was permitted this extensive latitude in observing the residents and the nursing staff, I became aware of the differences I have just described and was thus in a position to formulate the causes for it. Moreover, all these people, including the nursing staff, allowed me to forget my age and to utilize the fruits of many years of work in my personal and sometimes unorthodox manner. I owe to all of them the increase in my self-confidence and ability to clarify my concepts about the place and the function of the aged in our society. I also owe to them unlimited gratitude for enabling me to become living proof that old age does not need to mean resignation from life and abdication from critical thinking.

If I succeeded in fulfilling the aims I have set for myself in this study, I will feel that I have discharged the debt I incurred so many years ago, and that I have also justified the chance my superiors at the institute took by allowing me to become part of their team. I also hope that I will have helped other people to face their own prejudices against the aged and thus made it possible to overcome them. In my own attempts to get to know the aged better, I not only lost my prejudice but learned to appreciate them. Whatever positive I have been able to discover about the aged and am able to report about them has come from the aged themselves, who have proved it through their contribution to their contemporaries. Last, but by no means least, I trust that I have succeeded in giving hope to aged people and taught them that life does not need to be empty and dismal as the years pile up.

SUCCESSFUL AGING

One

A NEW "MINORITY"?

*M*any factors that enter into the negative attitude toward the aged—especially the psychological ones—need investigation and explanation if more than perfunctory improvement is to be achieved. It is obvious that much of the rejection of old people stems from prejudice. It is characteristic of human nature that we feel most comfortable with the familiar. When confronted with anything unknown or foreign, we have to overcome an involuntary flight reflex before we can make contact with it. And old age is something foreign to almost anyone who is younger, even if he has spent his childhood years in close contact with a grandparent or other aged relative.

Because such early contact is easily forgotten as time goes on, the mere idea of the existence of the aged, especially in large and ever-increasing numbers, is extremely upsetting to the people who have to deal with them as a group. The measures they take on behalf of the aged are evidence of the general reluctance to face them and their problems squarely.

HOW LAWS AND LAWMAKERS FAIL THE AGED

To illustrate the reality of the barrier that is maintained between the aged and the rest of the population, I would like to describe

1

the curious ways in which our legislators deal with this large portion of our population.

In 1972, Congress raised Social Security payments very generously; in 1973, in an effort to bolster the pride of the aged poor, it shifted responsibility for payments from local welfare departments to the Social Security system. Despite the good intentions behind these moves, many of the aged lost more from them than they gained. Neither measure took into consideration the concomitant Medicaid rule on eligibility. This federally supported health care is available only to people whose income is below a specified level. Since the Medicaid figure was not adjusted upward to retain coverage for those whose increased Social Security payments put them over this level, these aged had to rely solely on Medicare—another federal program designed to help old people of all income levels. But Medicare does not pay the costs of appliances—such as eyeglasses, hearing aids, dentures—that are vital to the aged. Those too poor to pay for them out of their own pockets were forced to do without.

One would assume that Congress arrived at its decision on these measures after lengthy and thorough research. It is inconceivable that these people were not aware of the fact that the increase would conflict in a large number of cases with eligibility for Medicaid. It is equally inconceivable that this turn of events was intended. We can only assume that these bills had motivations other than the welfare of the aged poor.

The omission in this bill (as originally written) of any adjustment of Medicaid limits to the new rates for Social Security benefits demonstrates clearly the ambivalent attitude of the general population toward the aged: giving with one hand and taking away with the other. The members of Congress, their aides, their experts, and the rest of the committee staffs who were involved in this decision comprise as good a cross section of the American population as one can find. They include people from all parts of the country, of all ages, both sexes, all professional levels, all religious denominations, and all political shades. The apparent thoughtlessness and ambivalence toward the aged in the legislation they produced underlie the plight of the old.

A great many people will deny these facts and cite the numerous improvements that have been and are being proposed by well-meaning politicians in Congress and the state legislatures. It is quite true that in many other aspects in the life of the aged, the federal government has taken the lead in proposing measures for the amelioration of their predicaments and needs. Unfortunately, ambivalence plays its tricks here also.

Many of these proposals have been voted into law. You can read about them often enough in the papers, especially just before election time, but in a great many instances this is where the matter ends. The laws are on the books, but no means are provided to implement them. There is either not enough trained personnel to set up the machinery or not enough money to run it; in some cases both are lacking. Nothing happens until a new law is passed—with a similar result.

And what is worse, when economy measures are contemplated, the first cuts proposed are in budgets that help the aged. Recently *The New York Times* reported that one of the service programs for the aged was threatened with discontinuance for lack of funds. At stake was an agency through which the aged render services for other aged—chores such as picking up groceries and cleaning for the immobile aged, delivering rent checks, and in some cases, just keeping them company. The workers earn an average of $35 a week for sixteen hours of work. The budget for this program in New York City is $200,000. Even if the funding can be found in the end, the uncertainty and the prospect of losing this small addition to his meager Social Security payments must be torture to anyone who is dependent on this salary—not to mention the hardship to those dependent on these services. On August 28, 1974, funds for this important project were finally assured, two years and five months after the project was started. The money came from ACTION, the Federal agency for volunteer services.

This halfhearted interest in the aged cannot be explained by politics alone. After all, the men and women who make the laws are humane and full of good will. Some of them are even in the age group they are supposed to be helping; some of them have parents who would benefit from more active efforts for their welfare. This is further proof that because of the all but ineradicable prejudice against the aged, the concern for them is not genuine. The steps taken by the people in power represent merely attempts to pacify their consciences. Constantly prodded by the advocates for the aged, they make promises—most of them unfulfillable—to quiet the petitioners. It is these promises that exasperate the people who ask for help and who get tired of waiting for implementation that never arrives. One becomes convinced that only a few of the legislators really care about the effectiveness of their own laws. Otherwise, they would not repeatedly pass laws without the means to put them into action. The veto that often comes from the higher-ups, in the name of economy, absolves them from feeling guilty. When actual improvements are made, they are done so almost reluctantly, even condescendingly, as if the old ought to be grateful for being given what is after all their due.

"WHAT SHOULD WE DO WITH MOTHER?"

Another example of the condescending attitude was an article published in one of the leading women's magazines several years ago, when the problem of aging had just begun to attract public attention. It was called "What Should We Do with Mother?" This title indicates that the problem existed then, as it does now. It is as if "Mother" is not a person who has a voice in the planning of her future, but some object that must be disposed of by the most efficient and unobtrusive means possible. A great many publications today are written from the same viewpoint. Statistics are compiled, tabulated, and analyzed without any regard for the fact that it is people who are being discussed. Similarly, the establishment of large residences for the aged is proof of the desire to have old people out of the way and yet not harm them too much in the process. Much is made of the advantages of old-age homes because of the special protective features they offer, such as ramps instead of stairs, but the effects on the individual of his physical and psychological isolation from the rest of the population are rarely taken into account.

All this shows that old people, by and large, no longer have the prestige and respect that was traditionally accorded them. If a young person has occasion to realize that an old person is holding his own, he acknowledges it with surprise and condescendingly. I experienced this same attitude many years ago when there were only a few women with a higher education. My achievement was usually acknowledged with a phrase like this: "Well, for a woman, you are doing all right." The same remark is repeated today: "Well, for an old lady, you're doing all right."

As a rule, old people are shoved aside as if contact with them carried contagion. When an old person shows strong emotion— whether anger or love—he is reproached and criticized: "He ought to know better." But the younger person feels no compunction against letting go whenever he feels like it.

FEAR OF THE UNKNOWN

It would be unfair to accuse younger people of ill will in their desire to keep the old person at a safe distance. Nor can one blame younger people for not trying to understand the older one and for not being more helpful because of their lack of understanding. Try as one may, no one can project himself into the future— neither his own nor anyone else's. We can understand the phases of human development that we all have been through: childhood, adolescence, and adulthood. However different we are from one another, there are certain situations we all share, at least enough to be able to put ourselves into the other person's shoes. If that were not the case, society could not exist; there would be no give and take and no communication among people. In *The Merchant of Venice*, Shakespeare expressed what it is like not to be able to project oneself into another's place:

> Hath not a Jew eyes? Hath not a Jew hands, organs, dimensions, senses, affections, passions? fed with the same food, hurt with the same weapons, subject to the same diseases, healed by the same means, warmed and cooled by the same winter and summer, as a Christian is? If you prick us, do we not bleed? if you tickle us, do we not laugh? if you poison us, do we not die? and if you wrong us, shall we not revenge?
>
> —Act III, Scene 1

If one substitutes the word "aged" for "Jew," and "the rest of the population" for "Christian," this describes the present-day position of the aged better than any scientific thesis. In other words, people can get along with each other as long as they are able and willing to project themselves into the situation of another person.

But one situation in life where this projection is impossible is the future. No one has become old and then young again and told us what it was like to be old. Nor can one compare being old with the experience of a young person who has been at the brink of death because of illness, and then returned to health (youth) again. There is a fundamental difference between the two situations: no matter how ill a young person may be and no matter how much he may suffer, there is always hope to keep up his spirits and to give him the strength to endure and overcome a crisis. In the process of getting old, there is no hope of turning back and no hope of retracing one's steps to renewed vigor and strength.

It is just as impossible to conceive what our own future will be like as it is to predict someone else's. You can readily test this statement by asking anyone what he thinks his life will be like twenty-five years from now. He will tell you about hopes and plans mapped out for a person of the age he is now, with no thought that he may feel different in another quarter of a century. In addition, people's plans for the future are, in many instances, pipe dreams, not intended ever to be realized. When the time comes for these fantasies and plans to be put into practice, physical, psychological, or economic obstacles may make them impossible to carry out. Then a great disillusionment frequently sets in, with consequences that may lead to emotional complications in the normal process of aging.

Our inability to project ourselves into our own future makes it impossible for younger people to have sufficient sympathy and understanding for old people. The young voice their resentment of the old in various ways: "Why aren't they glad to be alive; why do they have to make so many demands? It's time to make room at the top." Even when these feelings are not put into words, one can be certain they exist.

The one and only redeeming feature about our inability to project ourselves into the future is this: it is unthinkable that man could—or would want to—live out his life if his future were an open book. All we can do about the future is to prepare ourselves as well as we can to accept unexpected changes in our lives and either adapt ourselves to the new situation or look for ways in which to adapt the changed situation to our needs.

Aversion to the aged is not limited to the young; it is well-nigh universal, shared even by many who have to treat the aged professionally. A middle-aged colleague frankly admitted to me that when an aged patient consults him, he has to overcome a tendency to withdraw. He explained his reaction: "When I have a younger patient, I can usually do something for him. I do not have this chance so often with an old person." Although this man is a first-rate specialist, he has given up before he starts. This, however, is only part of the story. The rest can be expressed in the phrase "There, but for the grace of God, go I."

CHILDHOOD SOURCES OF RESENTMENT

There are many reasons for the conscious or unconscious rejection of the older generation. Early conflicts with parents and parent figures that are never completely resolved may recur to plague the relationship between the generations, just when the elder ones are most dependent on the younger. Attempts to overcome early conflicts may not be entirely successful and may result in the ambivalence I mentioned earlier. That is why no child, regardless of age, can tolerate his parent aging and growing feeble without accompanying guilt feelings.

FEAR OF DEATH AND THE DEAD

This terror is closely connected with the concept of one's own death, death itself, the dead, and anything that has to do with the approaching end. One must, therefore, in self-defense, stay away from anything close to this threat. Death itself represents the UNKNOWN—a cause of fear, since no one can ever know what happens afterward. The dead themselves are a threat and have always been, as proved by the manifold burial rituals that have been in use ever since civilization started. Primitive people and children believe in magic and are therefore superstitious. A great many adults, including some rather enlightened people, never outgrow this belief. The very attraction and the lasting popularity of Charles Dickens' *Christmas Carol* or Shakespeare's *Hamlet* testify to the fact that there is a grain of fear of the dead and of their power over the living in almost all of us. In the effort to ward off this threat, we refrain from even pronouncing the words, because there is magic in the words themselves. We recognize this when we say: "Speak of the devil. . . ."

If the topic cannot be avoided, we use circumlocutions in order not to provoke "reprisals." Old people are referred to by gentle euphemisms such as "elderly," "advanced in years," "senior citizens," "the golden-age group." The word "death" is circumvented with an array of synonyms: "passing away," "departure," "demise," "loss," and many others. The dread of contagion created by the proximity of old people expresses our fear of death, our fear of challenging fate, as though we will hasten the end of life if we call it by its proper name or associate with people who are near it.

This aversion is more unconscious than conscious, yet it is a powerful element of the ambivalence in the relationship of the younger to the old; of the self-depreciation of the old, and of the inertia that occurs whenever measures are to be taken on their behalf. There is one fallacy in this line of thinking: looking away from a problem does not solve it.

THE MINORITY WE CANNOT ESCAPE

All these mechanisms lead to a withdrawal from too close an association with the aged, to an effort to force the aged into the status of a social minority, though their numbers are growing constantly. Stratification of society has always existed; groups have been formed to unite people who share mutual interests as well as prejudices created by values the individual member acquired in childhood. By excluding "the outsiders," groups protect their own way of life and avoid contact with anyone whom they regard as different from themselves or inferior. The barriers raised against people of a given "race, color, or creed" have plagued mankind forever. And behind these barriers, people can retain their prejudices and organize their own lives in such a way that they have little or no contact with a group they do not like.

But no such isolation is possible in the long run in dealing with people in this minority—the aged. They penetrate every barrier, because they occur everywhere, regardless of "race, color, or creed." Everyone is bound to join their ranks sometime, and everyone is bound to become one of those shunned. This rejection continues even into old age and gives rise to self-hatred. It is in part due to that fact that the old one was one of those who did the rejecting not so long ago.

Last but not least, the relationship between the old and the young is greatly dependent on the younger one's attitude toward his own aging, his fear of death, of losing power and attractiveness. Fear of pain and illness plays a substantial part too.

ECONOMICS AND OLD AGE

For this study, aging has been investigated mainly from the medical and psychological standpoints. Yet economic circumstances also have considerable influence on the public attitudes toward old age. In an economy that as a rule discards old or nonfunctioning objects rather than repairing them, old or nonfunctioning people may be thought expendable as well. It is not considered very prudent to invest a great deal of money, time, or energy in something that does not promise to yield productive returns. This includes not only the aged but also people with incurable diseases, mental de-

fectives, and lawbreakers, who are jailed but are given little opportunity for rehabilitation. Any investment in people in these
categories serves mainly as a means of assuaging the guilt feelings
of those not yet afflicted.

THE AGED AGAINST THEMSELVES

The aged themselves must accept a good share of the blame for
society's neglect and lack of respect. A great many of them do not
make it easy for others to like them. To begin with, anyone old and
disheveled in appearance is bound to be less attractive than someone
young and well groomed. The behavior of an old person sometimes
shows him to disadvantage; he may be disgruntled, angry, even
hostile. Because of physical infirmities, he may not be able to
take care of his exterior the way he should, and sometimes he does
not even realize the degree of his physical neglect. In other words,
not every old person is lovable. Moreover, as I have said, the old
often hate themselves and take out their hatred on others.

As the impasse between the old and the young becomes wider
and wider, the ever-increasing number of aged makes the solution
of this problem more urgent every day. A bridge must be found
between the younger and older generations; otherwise we will have
to term the situation of the aged hopeless. There is, fortunately, a
psychological mechanism called empathy that some thoughtful people use whenever they are confronted with a human situation that
they have not experienced personally. Some people have a natural
faculty for understanding and relating to people they do not know
well. Yet a great many people hardly take this trouble; they simply
expect the other person to feel and think the same as they. If they
find that this is not the case, they have no use for him.

Several decades ago, some people endeavored to make a
special study of the psychic mechanisms of human beings; psy-

chiatry as we know it today is the result. It teaches its students first of all the concept of empathy. How else could a healthy and sane person know what a mentally disturbed person suffers and what agony he may go through? By anticipating the emotional turmoil, a psychiatrist can sometimes reach the mentally sick and open the way toward insight and recovery. When dealing with situations about which he can only guess, he applies the same ability to anticipate. And by guessing correctly what an old person feels and does not want to or is not able to put into words, he can make a bridge between himself and the oldster.

This is not easy to accomplish and demands a great deal of patience, but it has led to the beginning of a better understanding between some groups of adults and aged, and it will, I hope, lead to more give-and-take and to greater appreciation of each other.

Two

AGING

*W*hat is aging? Neither biology nor medicine can give an answer to this question. We can describe the signs of aging, we can understand the nature and the origins of the illnesses that occur mainly in the later years of our lives, but we do not know what aging is. We do know that signs of aging begin to appear in humans, as everywhere in nature, as soon as full maturity has been achieved. And like the process of maturing, aging does not take place at the same rate in every individual or in the same sequence or with the same intensity. The onset is gradual under normal conditions, more drastic and more rapid under stress.

Equally undefinable is another concept that is just as important to our investigation as the concept of aging, namely, normality. To illustrate this point: the weight of a person of a given height varies "normally" between a minimum and a maximum. Any variation below and above these approximations we term "abnormal." A similar approximation is involved when we speak of "normal" body temperature, "normal" blood pressure, etc. Many individuals have a "norm" that is higher or lower than the average, yet they are completely healthy. From this it follows that "health," too, is an approximation.

Once these concepts have been clarified, we can proceed to investigate the combination of these two postulates: normal aging.

This is the premise on which this book is based; it will enable us to measure and understand various manifestations of aging and to judge how close to or how far from these standards we are, and how much we can expect of ourselves as we get older and older.

After a long search for what I considered a scientific definition of the concept "health," I finally found an answer that seemed right—one that, with one qualification, seems also to comprehend the problem of healthy aging. It was formulated by Anthony Lenzer, associate professor of public health and human development at the University of Hawaii:

> Health is defined as the ability to function well enough to carry out normal roles and responsibilities in the community. This definition has several advantages. It is relatively easy to determine how well people are functioning; it directs attention to conditions within the individual or environment which, when corrected, will improve functioning; and, it makes sense to the aged, if not to the professionals.*

This would apply perfectly to healthy aging if it were not for one phenomenon that must be sharply separated from the concept of aging as such: this is the series of ailments that most often occur in later life. As long as an aging person is lucky enough not to be afflicted with illnesses that are painful or impair functioning, aging itself is not noticeable to him until it has become far advanced. This is why so many aged people will tell you that they do not feel any different from the way they felt when they were young.

Before proceeding, I would like to return to the statement on empathy that I made in the first chapter: that the faculty of empathizing is the basis for the differentiation between the mentally healthy and the mentally sick. And if this explanation does not satisfy the doubter, let me cite a statement by Sigmund Freud that

* "Health Care Services," in *Working with Older People* (Rockville, Md.: U.S. Department of Health, Education, and Welfare, May 1972), vol. 3, p. 63.

is one of the basic postulates of his theories: there are no qualitative differences between the well and the sick; there are only quantitative differences. That is, whatever goes on in the sick is to be found also in the well, only in a more moderate and better organized fashion.

Aging is the decline in functional capacity, lessened resilience, and increased vulnerability to disease. Every one of these manifestations is progressive and irreversible. Stress occurs when the person is exposed to undue demands on his energies that may be caused by illness, accident, or psychological impact (not necessarily severe in nature) that throw the body off balance, even if only temporarily. These undue demands can also arise from changes in the life situation of the individual.

THE SENSE ORGANS BECOME OLDER

What happens when the body becomes noticeably older? Since the contact of the individual with his external world is made through the sense organs, they seem the best point at which to start describing the aging process.

Failing eyesight is the first symptom that makes the individual aware of his advancing years. Reading glasses become necessary in the middle forties; not much later, stronger illumination is needed in order to see things clearly. Impairment of vision and the need to seek help, including surgery where necessary, are now commonly accepted, but the time is not long past when no female of any age would appear in public wearing glasses. A verse by the late Dorothy Parker explains this taboo:

> Men seldom make passes
> At girls who wear glasses.*

* "News Item" from *The Portable Dorothy Parker*, Copyright 1926, 1954 by Dorothy Parker, reprinted by permission of The Viking Press, Inc.

The prejudice implied in this bon mot has no age limit for quite a few women to this day.

The sense of hearing is the next to become duller. Diminution of hearing is not so easily discovered as impairment of vision, and even less readily admitted. Usually the people around the aging person notice the developing defect much earlier than he does, but are too timid or too tactful to draw attention to it. One reason that someone may be unaware that he has become hard of hearing is that even people with normal hearing guess quite a few sounds without realizing that they are guessing. The hard of hearing make wrong guesses more frequently—a fact that has often been exploited to create a humorous situation at the expense of the deaf person. Another reason for the resistance to admitting a hearing loss dates back to the time when the only available hearing aid was an ear trumpet; those who used them were often ridiculed and made ashamed of their inability to hear. With the application of electronics to the production of hearing aids, this objection to them is gradually diminishing, and most wearers obtain remarkable improvement in using them.

Taste and smell are also affected by aging, but their changes are less understood and appreciated. People who are in contact with the elderly will tell you that they have two major complaints—food and their children. The complaint about food is easily explained when one considers how the taste buds work. Distributed over the tongue, they last no longer than a few days each and then are replaced. In keeping with the general slowing-down process, they are renewed more slowly than they are used up. This means that the total number of effective taste buds declines, and, therefore, food tastes less savory. Extensive dentures that cover a large portion of the oral cavity diminish the perception of taste even further. In addition, there is the close interrelationship between smell and taste. Anyone who has ever had a cold can testify to the fact that while the cold lasts, not only is the sense of smell reduced, but food loses its taste as well. There is a similar deterioration in the sense of smell as a result of the process of aging.

The sense of touch and the position sense both lose a great deal of acuity as time goes on. For that reason, as well as because of changes in muscle sense and muscle strength—in both the voluntary and involuntary muscle groups—more exertion is needed to take a firm grip when carrying or handling objects. Consequently, older people drop things more often than they used to. The same effort that lifted a foot for safe walking is not sufficient in later years to produce the same action. The result is more frequent stumbling, falling, and subsequent fractures.

There is also a lessening of what we call the sense of balance. When changing position, for instance, from horizontal to vertical, we may feel a slight insecurity about our orientation in space. This lasts but a fraction of a second and occurs mostly when the motion is made rapidly. This short period, however, is often enough to cause loss of balance and a fall.

The perception of pain diminishes too, although in varying degrees with different people. Pain is a very important warning signal, and so is heightened body temperature; they announce the existence of something that is harmful to the body and needs medical attention. Both these manifestations are also subject to the general slowing-down process. A delay in perceiving them may permit an illness to progress to an advanced stage without being detected. To guard against this possibility, regular and thorough medical examinations should become routine in the life of every aged person.

The psychological deprivations resulting from the loss of acuity in the sense organs are no less important than the physical effects. Over the long period during which the loss takes place, the aged gradually stops missing familiar stimulations and sensations. This leads to more isolation and sensual impoverishment of the individual, who in turn responds to these deficiencies with further withdrawals. Just as anyone who was lucky enough to avail himself of successful remedial treatment, such as a cataract operation, will understand the ecstasy one feels when seeing color again in the natural state, so there is a parallel nostalgic pleasure when hearing again the raindrops on the window sill with the help of a newly acquired hearing aid. It is only then that an older person realizes how much he had lost through the deterioration of a sense organ, and he is grateful for the return of the world that he thought he had lost forever. This is one of the positive pleasures to be had in later life if one tries. Unfortunately, many an old person is too proud to admit to anyone, including himself, that he needs help; he does not even inquire whether any remedy is available.

OTHER FUNCTIONAL CHANGES

There are other physiological changes that every aging person has to contend with, although in different degrees. The blood circulation undergoes impairment, and so do the respiratory organs. It takes longer to catch one's breath after exertion, and a diminution of staying power sets in too. The tempo in which daily chores can be accomplished becomes slower and slower. More time is needed for the same activities; the schedule lags, and at the end of the day the older person feels exhausted without having accomplished what he had set out to do. As a result, he is frustrated and angry with himself.

Digestion and elimination are also affected by the aging process and are sometimes a source of embarrassment to a fastidious oldster.

The sex organs are not exempt from the aging process. In addition to their physical changes, their connection with the emotional aspects of our lives, as well as their social implications, is so crucial that I shall discuss this subject at length later on.

Although old skills remain unimpaired for a very long time, the ability to learn new material slows down perceptibly. Memory begins to fail, mostly in the ability to keep names and new concepts in mind for any length of time. The emotions become flatter. The time-honored assumption that the aged become more mellow and more tolerant is a myth; it simply means that they begin to care less. They have learned by painful experience that a great many things take care of themselves, if given time.

ILLNESS AND AGING

The aging process has been accused of causing the many prolonged illnesses that are prevalent among older people. It must be emphasized that this is not the case. Chronic illnesses begin to establish themselves in the organism much earlier, but for a long time they remain dormant, displaying no symptoms. I have in mind the various metabolic diseases, such as diabetes, stone formations, intestinal ulcers, arthritis. Other such illnesses are due to the changes that occur in the vascular system—among them, heart conditions, high blood pressure, hardening of the arteries, and many more. All these afflictions can be precipitated and aggravated by stress—including aging itself and its psychological impact on the aging person.

With the help of modern medicine, most of these prolonged illnesses do not present a threat to life. Yet some of them force the patient to follow a rigid diet or a special mode of living. The need to adhere to a restricted diet increases the discontent with food mentioned earlier. The person involved usually overindulged in the dishes that are now taboo, and he must now eat the things he never liked.

Some prolonged illnesses cause pain and diminished mobility, which force the individual to reduce his radius of action. When a small trip becomes a major project, it seems almost easier to remain at home.

The last vicissitude of old age is that most dreaded one, a malignancy. Here, too, medicine has come a long way. Early-detection methods—which make surgery, chemotherapy, and radiation the treatment of choice in a great many instances—can give the patient an extended lease on life. And even in cases where this would not have any lasting effect, there are now many means to keep suffering at a minimum and make this period of life more bearable. It may be reassuring to some of the aged to learn that the later in life the illness occurs, the less virulent its course usually is. Moreover, I am convinced that most old people suffering from a terminal disease fear the pain it may cause more than the illness.

EXTERNAL STRESS

The demands of life begin to intensify soon after the age of forty. A man may be concerned that the security of his job is in doubt; a woman whose children begin to leave home for school or a job or to get married finds her sphere of influence smaller. In addition, menopause, occurring approximately at this same period, is sometimes very discomforting, although fortunately only temporarily.

In the fifties, similar pressures occur, but to a greater degree, chiefly because of the impending early retirement with which various companies are experimenting. Until recently, the youth orientation of our country has been a threat only for people past sixty or sixty-five. But in many instances, the need to look for a new career or a new job actually begins around fifty or fifty-five; it is at fifty-five that some companies inform their executives whether they have any chance for future advancement.

But when the fateful year sixty-five rolls around and retirement becomes a reality, the pressures increase still further. By that time the physiological signs of aging have become noticeable, and so have the emotional responses they entail. Sources of special stress are the consequences of retirement, including forced idleness, lowered economic and social status, dislocation for economic reasons, a new job needing less skill and offering less pay; the disruption of the familiar social setting caused by death or the loss of old friends who had to move elsewhere.

All these changes represent psychological injuries whose effects are the same as those due to physical decline in the course of aging.

THE EMOTIONAL RESPONSES

As I have pointed out, man experiences the world through his sense organs. He understands its happenings through his intellect; he evaluates them with the help of his psyche. In this way, the psyche pervades whatever goes on within the individual. As a matter of fact, the way in which a person reacts to internal and external changes has a greater impact on him and his personality than the changes themselves. Consequently, the way a person deals with the manifestations of his aging can make him old ahead of time or can keep him young and spry, perhaps to the very end.

The first signs of aging are often ignored; later on, cosmetics, physical exercise, special diets, and other measures are resorted to, and with their help, the "moment of truth" can be postponed for quite a while. If these compensatory activities are overdone for any length of time, they accelerate the process of aging instead of retarding it. They demand the expenditure of more physical and psychic energy than can be restored through rest and relaxation. When that happens, many reasons (better called "rationalizations") are then advanced, such as illness, the wrong job, etc., to explain the rapid diminution of one's own effectiveness. But as in any failure, the self-respect suffers blow after blow, followed by guilt feelings, self-reproaches for falling down on the job, and subsequent self-hatred.

Chronic depression is rather frequent among the aged. A hearty belly laugh, which was so exhilarating in younger years, occurs only rarely. The sense of humor is greatly diminished in the old, and in the morning, they get up disgruntled because they did not sleep well. As a matter of fact, I am convinced that no old person is entirely free from at least occasional depressions.

Depression in old age differs from that in youth in one respect, however. In the aged, the anger is directed more against the person himself than against anyone in the outer world.* This self-hatred and self-rejection explain in part the high rate of suicide among the older generation.

In order to preserve what is left of their self-esteem, old people establish many defenses. Anxiety and variability of mood are frequently employed to keep family and friends on their toes. However, some anxiety is to be expected; a certain degree of concern about health is natural for any aging person since his power of resistance to illness and injury is actually diminished. This holds true for dependency also. No older person, try as he may, is able to manage completely by himself as easily as a younger person. Small chores around the house have to be left undone because of the risk involved; for instance, one cannot and should not climb a ladder or lift heavy weights. This increased dependency on assistance represents at times a burden for others, especially if the

---

* Robert H. Dovenmuhle, *Aging in Modern Society*. Psychiatric Research Reports of the American Psychiatric Association, Report no. 23, ed. Alexander Simon and Leon J. Epstein (New York: American Psychiatric Association, 1967–68), pp. 81–87.

aged person utilizes his need to be helped as a means of getting attention.

Even if these attention-getting devices are successful, the aged person is only momentarily satisfied. The more unnecessary assistance he gets, the more helpless he will become, and before long he will have become so infantilized that the aging process will be hastened, not relieved. If the aged and the people in his environment receive proper education on this danger, wonders can be accomplished.

Another defense mechanism employed by many old people is the "process of disengagement" (a term coined by Elaine Cummings and William E. Henry). With the ability to lead their former busy life diminished, they quite naturally must make a selective reduction in their activities. If the individual continues to be involved with his remaining interests as much as he was before, this is "normal disengagement." If he withdraws from his contacts with the world and people, concentrating solely on himself and simply waiting for death, this would have to be called "unwholesome disengagement."*

There are real factors that make the old person feel that the world is turning against him. There is a widening gap between the aged, his habits, standards, skills, and "modern ways." He feels and is made to feel antiquated and out of place; he gradually becomes aware of the rejection by, and almost contempt of the younger generation for most of the accomplishments and ideas that were dear to him throughout his life. In addition, his general decline, which prevents him from keeping pace with the rapid tempo of change, reinforces his insecurity and anxiety. He prefers to retreat into his shell. But while it seems that the aged is withdrawing

---

* *Growing Old: The Process of Disengagement* (New York: Basic Books, 1961), p. 61.

from the world, in fact it is the world that is withdrawing from him or, if you prefer, casting him out. In their desire to remain independent, old people become recluses; they turn away entirely from the environment and the people they used to know. We find this type on all levels of society—in large, old-fashioned mansions and in walk-up apartments, living in disorder, filth, and suffering from various kinds of physical neglect, including malnutrition. This is the mechanism of withdrawal to a pathological degree— unwholesome disengagement. It is caused by false pride, lack of information about available facilities, and misinterpretation of the manifestations of aging.

The consequence of this withdrawal is that the world around the oldster furnishes less stimulation than it used to; the satisfactions that come from outside become poorer. He therefore looks to his past for his satisfactions. This explains the tendency to idealize days gone by, unconsciously omitting the unpleasant aspects and emphasizing the favorable side. The world he now remembers was one where he was somebody who counted, where he felt more at home and more comfortable than in the strange new world. As a matter of fact, the "good old days" weren't so good at the time they happened as they are in the minds of the ones who remember them. If left to himself, this way of thinking may eventually lead to more serious mental disorders, but with the help of proper medication and family therapy, the aged may make better contact with the present.

EFFECTS ON PERSONALITY

Contrary to general belief, old age does not produce fundamental changes in the personality. Everyone acquires his psychic mechanisms in early childhood and repeats them in the face of new situations and problems that subsequently arise. The problems confronting the person in old age are no exception. His particular characteristics may intensify, timidity and dependency may increase, but the problems have increased also. When we notice an old person showing hypochondriacal tendencies, we have a right to assume that he has always been concerned with his health but has kept his concern hidden from his friends. The opposite may also occur. Some people deny any illness and belittle any discomfort in order to keep the image they have of themselves as strong and self-reliant. Actually, this "escape into health" may be just a camouflage for the fear of death.

When personality traits of a specific nature appear, such as quarrelsomeness or a suspicion of being robbed or otherwise taken advantage of, we must be prepared to find other signs of a serious mental decline. But there must be more than one symptom before we can come to such a conclusion. Suspiciousness alone would not be astonishing. We must remember that memory begins to weaken in everyone who is advancing in years, and he simply forgets where he put things. It is but a step to the suspicion of being robbed. Quarrelsomeness may be closely connected with physical pain and perpetual frustration, understandable complaints in this age group.

An additional characteristic that is particularly attributed to "personality changes" in old age is a gradual trend toward economy in spending, up to the proverbial miserliness. I believe that this character trait is gradually lessening among people getting older today.

The present-day aged were imbued in childhood with the idea that they should leave something to their children after their death. Coupled with the self-hatred of so many aged persons, the idea of spending anything more than absolutely necessary becomes abhorrent. They continue wearing their old clothes and eat the cheapest food and put their savings under the mattress.

It is quite surprising to observe that the younger among the aged, those who grew older since the enactment of Social Security and the loosening of family ties, are much more ready to live less frugally and do not begrudge themselves enjoyment in their old age. They are quite prepared to spend all the resources they have for their own comfort.

It was not very pleasant to write this chapter, because nobody likes to come face to face with his own decline. But it is time to remind my readers that what actually takes place in our bodies is not so important as what we make of it. And the way to get command over one's own foibles and weaknesses will be shown in the next chapter.

Three

SELF-ACCEPTANCE

*T*he changes that take place as we get older occur so gradually that they largely escape our notice. As long as a person remains physically well, he is hardly conscious of the passage of time. "I don't feel any different from the way I've always felt all my life," a friend in his sixties said when I asked him how he had first realized that he was getting older.

From his earliest days, a child is made aware that he is getting older; eventually he learns, to his great dismay, that this means displeasure, rejection, and renunciation. The small child who wants to be spoon-fed by Mama is told he is too old for that; he must use the spoon himself. When he wants to be carried, he is made to walk; and if he does not want to go to school while a younger brother remains at home with Mother, he is told that he's too old to stay at home. These denials—especially if there is a younger sibling who continues to enjoy these longed-for privileges —give the child the feeling of not being loved enough, of being rejected. He may also conclude that getting older is undesirable and unpleasant.

There are countless examples to show that many children dread growing up; actually the number who resist the maturing process is much larger than one might assume. It will be these children who will have more difficulties adjusting to their new status as old people than the ones who wanted to grow up. It is also small wonder that when they are old, they feel the same way and accept the widespread rejection due to their age as something that in childhood they had experienced as a part of life.

HOW AGING BEGINS

The diminution of physical prowess is the first hint of aging for both sexes, but it is especially noticeable in young men. Top performances in all the branches of athletics are age-bound. As a rule, a sprinter older than the early twenties is a rarity, and a heavyweight boxer in his early thirties has little chance of winning. The techniques of training athletes have improved considerably in recent decades so that the turning point for champions has been postponed for a few years, but not very many.

Cultural development, too, has been kind and prolonged the period in which men and women can be young. At the time that the present-day aged were young, an unmarried woman in her middle twenties was called an old maid. This was a period when most women did not receive sufficient education to enable them to enter the labor market. Getting married was the only way to secure protection in old age, unless the woman was content to end her life as a "poor relative" or, more accurately, an unpaid servant in the house of a more fortunate member of the family. When a woman reached thirty, she was considered to have joined the ranks of the middle-aged. Nowadays, young people mature earlier and stay young longer. Nevertheless—Women's Lib notwithstanding—it is still true that a woman who has not married by her middle twenties may become concerned that she will never get a husband. Even if she does not seem to care, her aging and old-fashioned parents do and will exert pressure on her to seek the haven of matrimony and live protected while raising a family. Since women have begun to embark on careers of their own, the "dangerous" age has moved from thirty to forty and even later, and women often retain a great deal of sex appeal many years longer.

THE MOMENT OF TRUTH APPROACHES

The first tell-tale signs occur when a man in his twenties begins to lose his hair, and both sexes grow some gray hair in their thirties. In spite of continuous physical exercise, the bodies of both sexes begin to show some flabbiness; "middle-aged spread" makes it necessary to buy clothes one or two sizes larger.

Aging usually becomes noticeable to those around you before it does to you yourself. The inroads the years make can be illustrated by self-observation: on a bus or subway, a young and attractive female may be offered a seat by both younger and older men. A few years later, while she may still be very attractive, she will find that only the older men demonstrate this gallantry. A few years later still, she may, to her surprise, be given a seat by a young girl. But when the time comes that she is offered a place by a middle-aged woman, she knows that she has reached old age.

Men have their warning signals too. When a man finds that he needs a second martini before he can enjoy dinner or a cat nap before he can be sociable after work—these are hints that times are changing. Or he may be looking appreciatively and flirtatiously at a young girl only to discover that she prefers his teen-age son. Or when leaving an elevator, a young subordinate may step aside to let him get off first. More seriously, he may be severely jolted by the news of a contemporary's heart attack.

Men and women with families are more age-conscious than childless couples and unmarried people. The reason is that they see their children become adults right before their eyes. The person without children continues much longer without the realization that time is running on. Some parents actually look forward to having their growing children leave home. After the last one has left, parents are often young enough to remake their lives together anew.

Beginning with World War II, marriages were entered into earlier and earlier, and the children arrived at a time when the parents had hardly reached physical and mental maturity. Stepping from school, military service, or apprenticeship into marriage and parenthood deprived the young couple of fun and the opportunity to abandon themselves occasionally to unbridled pleasure. As a consequence, in time to come, these parents tacitly encouraged their children to branch out on their own at a relatively early age. Thus the parents eventually regained the chance they had missed in their courtship or early marriage. The various combinations of sexual and social experimentation that the middle-aged are currently engaging in represent attempts to make up for lost time or to hold on to youth.

When the children leave home, a large number of women nowadays return to the calling for which they were trained and which they gave up for the sake of child-rearing. It is at the same time, in the early or middle forties, that many men, realizing that they have no chance for future advancement, leave their jobs. If a man has not been able to find his niche by that time, he may encounter difficulties locating a new position that is satisfactory or be forced to go into business for himself. This brings to mind President Franklin Roosevelt's plea to employers during the Depression to reserve some jobs for men over forty. Later on, when a man is in his fifties, it may not be easy to make a fresh start. These decisions, which offer great challenges for individuals in their forties, begin to slacken off in the fifties and early sixties, until old age takes us by surprise. As we have seen, the clues are innumerable, but most often they go unheeded unless a chronic illness forces attention to the changing state of affairs.

CAMOUFLAGE

According to Dr. Howard P. Rome, former president of the World Psychiatric Association, Americans spent $5 billion in 1970 for beauty aids, while the government spent $1.86 billion for old-age assistance in the same year. Would everyone not wish the figures were reversed? Tragically, much of the expenditure for cosmetics can be attributed to the enormous efforts people in a youth-oriented society make to improve their appearance and to hide the signs of aging. Dr. Rome's figure covers only outlays for "lotions, unguents, hair dyes, and cosmetics."* Not included in the $5 billion are the additional millions of dollars that are annually invested in cosmetic surgery: faces are lifted (a procedure that has to be repeated every two or three years), noses are remodeled, double chins are removed, rings under the eyes are eliminated, protruding ears are pinned back, and bosoms are made smaller or larger according to the builds and wishes of their owners. If only a portion of the money spent on these endeavors would be laid aside for the later years of life, a great deal of unhappiness, want, and misery could be prevented.

Sometimes the situation becomes pathetic when a person, usually a woman, does not know when to stop the attempts at rejuvenation. Hair dye covers the gray hair; face creams, rouge, and massages are applied, supposedly to make the skin of the face keep pace with the youthful hair coloring. Unfortunately, nature is not easily fooled. As the hair becomes gray, age also takes its toll on the skin. The elastic fibers that lie within the layers of the skin keep the facial expression lively, mobile, and expressive. As a person ages, the texture of the skin ages with him, and these elastic fibers especially slacken in their tensile strength in the

---

* Introductory remarks, by Howard P. Rome, M.D., *Psychiatric Annals*, *Geriatrics*, Part 1, vol. 2, no. 10 (October 1972), 7–11.

same way as a rubber band does after it has been used too long. The next resort is more make-up, which, in turn, contrasts more sharply with the crow's-feet around the eyes and thus produces the exact opposite of the effect intended; the dyed hair only makes the contrast more dramatic. Although fewer men use beauty aids to any great extent, the ever-increasing numbers of male beauty boutiques show that they have a fair share in the efforts to stay young. Shoulder-length white hair, thinning on top, is not attractive on an elderly man; neither is a miniskirt or pants on an elderly woman. Unfortunately, one not infrequently sees examples of this in both sexes. Folk humor is sometimes a harsh judge. A German saying— "A schoolgirl from the back, a mummy from the front"—indicates that the reluctance to accept aging is not confined entirely to the youth-oriented United States, as some experts would have us believe.

An aged person looks his or her best in an outfit that is tasteful and in harmony with the times as well as with his age. Some up-to-date adaptations are acceptable to show that one is aware of the changes in the environment. And if these modifications are employed discreetly, they will enhance the general appearance. One does not have to be rich to make oneself presentable, and simple means will usually suffice.

PSYCHOLOGICAL REPERCUSSIONS

As we accumulate experience in our personal development and in our skills, our performances and interests grow and widen, increasing our pride and self-esteem, as well as the status we have attained within our community. As the middle years come along, the pace of this development becomes slower until a certain plateau is reached. This fact ought to be the first signal of aging, but it is usually ignored or explained away by unrelated circumstances.

But when the slackening of the tempo and the diminution of our bodily functions can no longer be disregarded, the individual begins to torment himself with reproaches for falling down on the job. Although he may increase his efforts in order to keep up his usual tempo, he actually is faced with more and more frustrations and disappointments, which, in turn, create more self-hatred and feelings of guilt. Depression often occurs for the same reasons. During sleepless hours, every act of omission and commission comes back; every hurt suffered, justly or unjustly, every unpleasant incident returns to memory with heightened intensity. An old man who still functioned very well in his work confided to me: "At night I think of all the things I should have done and did not do."

One fact adds insult to injury because of its daily repetition, and that is the shock every old person gets when he looks at himself in the mirror in the morning. As we know, most old people will tell you that they do not feel old and that they feel as they always did. Looking into the mirror, they expect to see a picture that corresponds to the way they feel—young. What they actually see is the reflection of an old person who may be well preserved and, when smiling—as we usually do when we look at ourselves in the mirror—appearing perhaps younger than his age, but old just the same. This daily experience is a shock from which it is hard to recover. Some old people remove every mirror from their houses in order not to be reminded of the passing of time.

It bears repeating that each aged individual is depressed, at least part of the time. Some of the aged respond with more serious upsets that require special attention. On close scrutiny, one will find that these people have reacted to crises in the past in a similar manner, but usually with less intensity. This time the realization of the irrevocability of the process of aging, perhaps coupled with a prolonged and painful illness, has strained their ability to tolerate a major stress. After appropriate medical attention and assistance in the reorganization of their modes of living, they may make good, permanent adjustments. It is only a small percentage of the aging population that reacts so strongly to the changes in their lives. We must remember that they do not all occur at the same time and not in all people with the same intensity.

SELF-ACCEPTANCE BEGINS

Many people begin now to question the necessity of self-torture, because living has turned into just that. Little by little, the feeling of relief one gets from defaulting on some of the habitual demands of living becomes so satisfying that more and more experiments in this direction may be made. You may begin with an afternoon off from work, or a vacation that was previously considered extravagant and find that—to your great surprise—the world has not come to an end as a result. I asked a seventy-five-year-old man who is still very active in his business to describe the point at which he discovered he was getting old. He said: "It was two years ago, when I began taking taxis to the office instead of the subway." Another replied to the same question: "When I realized I had to go to the dentist more often." A third said: "When rheumatism started to plague me." None of these men expressed the thought that there was any lessening of his efficiency or of his interest in life.

It may be surprising that most of this testimony on how it feels to be old comes from men. Although quite a few men will admit to their age, they will insist, even in their seventies, that they feel as young as ever. But there are very few women indeed who will admit that they feel that they are getting on in years. As a matter of fact, they stop counting their years at forty or maybe fifty, and therefore can never admit that the years are adding up—much less that they feel old age coming on. I inquired once of a woman whom I knew to be sixty-nine how she felt about this topic, and she answered: "I am too young to give that idea any consideration." A seventy-five-year-old childless widow replied: "I will say something horrible. I do not like to be with old people. All they do is complain about their ailments." This woman has been seriously ill recently and has been trying very hard—but without success—not to complain. These last two examples show clearly the methods used in the denial of reality. The first one refused even to consider the problem posed to her; the other showed her self-rejection by projecting her prejudice onto the outside world.

Occasionally, one hears a sensible acceptance of reality, as in this statement by a seventy-six-year-old woman: "I don't mind getting older. I have fewer responsibilities, and I don't have to prove anything any more to anybody."

LEARNING TO APPRECIATE PHYSICAL COMFORT

The next step in self-acceptance may be enjoyment of physical comfort, such as a nap in the afternoon before going out in the evening, which turns out to be extremely rewarding. As the self-confidence grows, one even dares to defy the rules of fashion, for instance, by wearing comfortable shoes instead of the prescribed evening footwear. Suddenly one finds that there is no criticism even from the social arbiter of the group, because she, too, is getting on in years, and *her* feet also are beginning to hurt her. Actually, the rebel is admired for having the courage to put comfort above convention. In short, the sensible aged person begins more and more to assert himself instead of playing follow the leader. In the process of accepting himself, he ceases to be overwhelmed by the things he can no longer do. Finally, he questions why some of the usual chores that have accumulated over the years have become so burdensome, while others have not. He realizes that the burdensome jobs are the ones he really never wanted to do. By making a new inventory of the work to be done, he can streamline his daily routine and thus save energy. All of a sudden, life has become easier; he accomplishes more in the remaining areas than ever before. The motto now is: "I do not *have* to."

The guilt feelings about falling down on the job and the grieving about things one can no longer do are supplanted by a strong feeling of pride in the things one can still do. The same conscientiousness that had been invested in the many former activities, interests, and chores is now applied to the voluntarily restricted fields of activity; the same fastidiousness in appearance is maintained as before, only on a sensible scale. Liberation from a great many "oughts" that are no longer gratifying allows all the energies to be concentrated on the things one *wants* to do and enjoys doing.

BENDING WITH THE STORM

Some people are able to reach these conclusions by themselves, some need the help of trusted friends, and still others seek the assistance of a psychiatrist. Whatever the means, the moment arrives when the aged person realizes the futility of a struggle he cannot win. If this realization leads to acceptance of the inevitable, the effect is almost miraculous. The beauty aids are reduced to a bare minimum, the gray hair is accepted—at first reluctantly, later with pride—and the harmony between age and appearance is about to create a new individual. Insomnia abates, and depression occurs only occasionally. Self-esteem has been restored, and the person who has all but retired from life is ready to start anew and get as much out of it as he can.

Now that self-acceptance has supplanted self-hatred, there is no further need to expend psychic and physical energy in trying to turn back the clock; there is no need to waste strength in trying to keep pace with the young. Instead, there is an adaptation to what is left and to what it is possible to accomplish in proper proportion to the body's ability to restore the energies that are spent from day to day. In this way, your self-esteem comes into its own, and so does the courage to live. This newly acquired philosophy of life is suddenly reflected in your demeanor and in your whole personality; the over-all impression is more energetic, and your face and posture show less fatigue and less deterioration. What beauty aids cannot accomplish, peace of mind does. This new outlook is by no means to be interpreted as self-indulgence. It simply substitutes one set of values for another that is more workable at this stage of life.

Because the signs of aging accumulate little by little over a long period, it often takes only a small incident to precipitate the moment of self-acceptance. A man in his sixties observed that his moment came "when I stopped resenting anyone helping me put on my coat." He continued: "I now prefer sitting in an armchair because I can hold on to the arms of the chair when I get up. And if I know a woman well, I do not get up each time she enters the room." These concessions, and the equanimity with which this courtly Southerner related them, show that he had accepted himself while his pride and self-esteem remained intact. It is more than coincidental that he still follows his calling with the same vigor and intensity as always.

The struggle and the agony that a great many people undergo as they begin to realize that they are getting on in years have been expertly enumerated by Simone de Beauvoir in her book *The Coming of Age*. I do not feel adequate to pass judgment on the painstaking research evident in it. I can simply give my impression of the tenor of the book. One can only venture to guess the age group of the people described in this classic and what they went through in the process of the advance of their years. None of them, including the author herself, has progressed to the state of self-acceptance that alone can help master the misery and liberate the old person for new fields of interest, that can make him welcome new challenges. It is to be hoped that Madame de Beauvoir will reach this stage before long and give us an equally fine study of "Old Age Defeated."

By the time a person has reached the last third of his life span, he has learned that everyone has to make concessions and compromises in order to live peacefully. This last period, however, demands more of both than were necessary in younger years. Bending with the storm is the simplest way of diminishing its impact. Self-acceptance is just that. As long as the person enjoys moderately good health and is not burdened by too much pain, weathering the various storms successfully is relatively easy.

COPING WITH ILLNESS—REAL AND IMAGINED

There are, however, quite a few people who are not so fortunate in escaping debilitating pain—those who suffer from chronic diseases in addition to getting old. Sometimes, prolonged diseases demand more compromises than it is possible to make. What can people in this situation do to continue to enjoy living in spite of their suffering? Education can be a great help. Too many people still cling to the outmoded concept that old age is a disease in itself. The adherents of this theory stoically accept the developing infirmities as unavoidable. This is not true. In recent years a new medical branch called rehabilitation medicine has developed. It specializes not only in the treatment of prolonged diseases but also in assisting those afflicted with them to reorganize their lives in such a way that their handicap, if it cannot be cured, will hamper their activities as little as possible and, therefore, make living less painful. Too few of our aged—and, for that matter, too few of the general population—know about this new field of medicine and, consequently, fail to avail themselves of its services.

Some people cannot accept the fact that they are getting older and look for real and imaginary illnesses in order to explain the normal slowing down of their functions and to allay their own anxieties about aging. Afraid to learn the truth—whether encouraging or discouraging—they avoid seeking competent professional advice. Instead, they listen to a neighbor or a friend who has "been through the same thing." Rich or poor, they take refuge in patent medicines or cures peddled by high-pressure salesmen and fritter away money they often cannot spare on methods that cannot help them. I do not know what can be done on their behalf except to continue to try to convince them and their families that there are more accredited and more effective ways of getting help.

To summarize: I must emphasize that self-acceptance is fundamentally different from self-indulgence. Self-acceptance is the result of a common-sense appraisal of one's faculties, advantages, and disadvantages. Self-indulgence involves self-pampering and looking for excuses to be taken care of by others instead of making use of the assets that a person still commands. Through the second course, the individual becomes a burden not only to the people in his environment but also to himself, which makes the last stages of his life more painful than need be. On the other hand, self-acceptance leads to the diminution of guilt feelings and of feelings of inadequacy; it leads to lessening of tension and subsequent increase in psychic and physical energy. It also opens new avenues of self-expression that may make the last part of one's life more gratifying and more pleasant than one ever dreamed it could be.

Four

MAKING A NEW START

BUSINESS RELATIONSHIPS

As a person changes with the increase of his years, his role in life and his relationship to the people in his environment change too. While he and they mature and grow in their jobs, their paths are usually upward. His place among his contemporaries and the friends who grew up with him becomes more and more firmly established; in short, he belongs. But now that he has reached old age, he may suddenly be forced to face quite a few new facts, each of which comes as an unwelcome jolt. At work, the longtime colleagues are becoming fewer and fewer. They are retiring, moving away, dying. The vacancies thus created are filled by members of the younger generation who have much less personal knowledge of our old man and of his past achievements. And as the product of another period of our culture, this later generation is much less impressed by age, experience, reputation, and similar fruits of a long career.

Suddenly, long before retirement, the older person finds himself isolated, less important, less revered, and less self-confident as he sees the various props to his self-esteem disappear one by one. Finally, he feels antiquated and obsolete. If he is to retain proper mental and emotional balance, he will have to undertake a great deal of self-appraisal and self-acceptance.

SOCIAL RELATIONSHIPS

The downward curve is not confined to professional or business life; it encompasses the social aspect as well. A wife is now exposed to a similar experience in her own circle of friends. Gradually, at social gatherings, she ceases to be treated as an equal, as she had been in times past. She is now given the place of honor as an elderly dowager by hostesses who consider themselves to be younger (or younger-looking) than she is. She finds a gap between herself and the wives of her husband's younger associates; it will widen when her husband retires, and with more or less subtlety, she will be made to realize that her retired husband has lost his importance for the advancement of a former assistant.

Should she be widowed, her social standing may plummet even lower. It is banal, but nonetheless true, to observe that an un-attached woman, which she has now become, is not regarded as a social asset, while an unattached man—whatever his age—is always at a premium.

None of this is news to the person who has reached the last third of his life, since he himself, while on the other side of the fence, has probably been guilty of similar omissions and discriminations against his elders. He may even have considered such actions justified—as long as they concerned somebody else. What is news to him is that now it is he who is the subject of these same slights and discriminations. The near-aged who are often so thoughtless and unfeeling toward their elders seem unaware that the time when they in turn will be slighted is not so far off as they pretend.

THE DENIAL OF AGING

The realization that "this is happening to me" is the hardest fact for an aging person to own up to. Actually, old people do not feel any different from the way they always did and are sometimes quite taken aback when others refer to their getting older. On more than one occasion, I have made myself rather unpopular with some older people whom I knew only casually by asking them at what age they felt old and what circumstances made them feel so. Some of the answers have already been quoted, but here are some more: "I don't feel old at all," or, "I have to remind myself from time to time that I'm not getting younger."

Recently at a social gathering I asked that question again. One woman, very spry and lively at eighty-four, answered: "I felt old when I was given less work to do." All her adult life, she explained, she had been active in one charity organization and spent many years serving it in an executive capacity. Her co-workers evidently had noticed her slowing down and decided to ease her workload.

Another woman, who was sixty-five, at first denied that she felt old—except, as she phrased it, that she had less to do of late: "All I have to do is to look after myself and my husband. The children are all married and on their own."

I got a wholly divergent answer from a man who was in his early seventies. He emphatically denied that he felt any different from the way he had at thirty and cited as proof the fact that he still played tennis whenever he had the opportunity and skied during the winter.

These different responses all tell the same story: they are attempts to dissociate oneself from the unwelcome truth that aging is taking place. The attitude of each represents a defense mechanism that varies only in the intensity with which it denies reality. In support of people who successfully keep themselves from the realization that they are getting older, I must say that I agree with those of you who claim that you do not feel any different. An aging person feels old only at some moments and periods of unexpected fatigue—unexpected because he has forgotten to stop before his energies have become exhausted, as he should have anticipated.

LEANING AND BEING LEANED ON

Time has not stood still, and age has been taking its toll all around. Even if you remain healthy and feel as well as ever, some of your old friends have died or moved to other localities; your circle of contemporaries has begun to thin out.

With the narrowing of these human contacts, the aging person becomes more and more aware of the need to lean on some person or a group of peers. This is not a new manifestation but only a new realization that this fact exists. Beginning with birth, man must lean and depend on someone if he is to survive. He leans first on his mother; later, on his father, siblings and other members of the family, and his friends; still later, on his spouse. He does not think about these dependencies; they are more or less implied in the concept of interpersonal relationships. He is not conscious of this need to lean as well as to be leaned on. As a matter of fact, if anyone wanted to define what we call normal psychological maturity, one of the most important elements to be taken into account would be the ability to depend on and be depended on in return. Without this mutuality, normal adjustment to life cannot take place. This faculty is so important and plays such a large role in our existence that we are not aware of how indispensable it is for a well-balanced way of life.

As a man gets older, he necessarily loses some of his props, and he must look for new ones to keep going. If his family life has been successful, he will find these supports in his mate and grown children. Yet he may be dismayed to learn that he is in the process of losing his ability to be leaned on. This realization may well contribute to his depression and self-hatred, his low opinion of himself, and his increased loneliness.

In this connection, I would like to tell every old person this: if you feel downhearted because you cannot reciprocate the assistance you receive from your friends and family who are younger and stronger than you, you are making a great mistake. The way you are growing old will determine how your friends feel about you. If you have kept your self-esteem and your dignity, if you have remained interested in your friends and what is going on in the world, and if you have continued to participate in the lives of those who are still around, your contribution to the mutual support is equal to what you receive.

Margaret Blenkner* describes this dependency in old age "as a state of being, not a state of mind; a state of being in which to be old . . . is to be dependent. Such dependency is not pathological; it is not wrong; it is, in fact, a right of the old, recognized by most, if not all, societies."* This truth, as simply and sympathetically formulated, speaks for itself and ought to ease the mind of many an old person.

RETAINING INDEPENDENCE

Dependency on the younger generation will be more ideological than real, as long as health permits. In order to feel secure, one requires not so much the actual assistance as the knowledge that help will be there in case of need. Once the old one has this certainty, he will prefer independence for himself and his family; he will prefer to live his own life instead of being physically sheltered at the expense of his self-determination and freedom. He probably will voluntarily take second place and give the right of way to the younger ones, thus retaining his own self-respect and the respect of those who come after him.

This can best be accomplished by actively seeking new ties,

* "The Normal Dependencies of Aging," in *The Dependencies of Old People,* Occasional Papers in Gerontology, no. 6 (Ann Arbor: Institute of Gerontology, University of Michigan and Wayne State University), p. 27.

preferably among contemporaries. One does not form friendships easily at such a late date in life, but one can meet other lonely people and befriend them. Man is not made to live alone, and if he does, he pays a high price for it in the form of premature decline, either physical or mental or both. The need for companionship is probably one of the reasons that the new kinds of communal living among the aged have become so popular in such a short span of time. It is these expressions of inner freedom that will make the old one dearer to his family, and their devotion will be voluntary, not forced. It will also make it easier for the oldster to ask for advice if faced with a situation he cannot handle.

It is only the weak person with too little self-esteem who is too proud to ask for help, and who is afraid of losing face when he admits his need for assistance. In the same way, it is compatible with self-acceptance to ask for help when needed.

This kind of dependency must be sharply differentiated from pathological dependency. While the former always involves interaction and mutuality between the two parties, and while the roles are usually interchanged, a pathological dependency is always entirely one-sided. Its purpose is to get attention, assistance, and reassurance beyond the normal need without giving anything in return; it appears in people who, throughout their lives, have depended on the good will and the assistance and sympathy of other people without feeling indebted in any way. I can recall an old woman who had known better days and who was supported in her old age by friends of her family. She accepted their support as if it were her due. These people had paid her rent for many years. When the building she lived in was converted into a cooperative, they were not in a position to buy her apartment for her. This she took as a rejection and let the world know about their desertion.

In sharp contrast to this kind of dependent behavior is the life a friend of mine leads. The childless widow of a physician, she is now in her late seventies. While her husband was alive, they both ran a school for the training of medical secretaries. After his death she continued teaching at the school, until a very painful bone condition began to impair her mobility rather seriously. She gave up the school but continued teaching by writing textbooks on the subject, which have since become classics in the field.

In spite of her difficulties in getting around and the great pain she suffers with every step, she has never stopped being interested in her friends, who live not only in her home town but all over the globe. A few years ago she took a trip around the world to visit her far-flung circle. She arranged to be met with a wheelchair at the various airports en route. These friends and the ones who live nearby remain in touch with her, and she exchanges visits with them frequently. At no time does one hear a word of complaint—unless one asks a direct question. One cannot help but admire this indomitable spirit and the example she sets for her contemporaries in making the best of the time that is left for her in spite of her serious handicap.

REMAKING LIFE ON YOUR OWN

One of the most profound needs for readjustment in later life arises after the death of a mate. Marriages that have lasted for several decades create a kind of symbiosis between a husband and wife. They need not communicate verbally to know what the mate wants or needs at the moment. They also do not have to talk a great deal if issues are at stake, because, in the course of time, they have become familiar with each other's views. If one of them wants to remember something far in the past, he simply will ask the other. This togetherness does not necessarily mean that they have lived serenely with each other all these years; it simply means that the mere presence of the other is reassuring, even in an argument.

This mutual leaning and being leaned on is so much taken for granted that the loss of one mate by death creates a crisis of intense magnitude for the survivor. The shock can be so severe that it can break down even physical defenses. Only recently it has become known that bereavement in later years can precipitate physical illness, such as diabetes and other afflictions of the organ system, by diminishing the natural resistances against illness and the will to live. This explains the increased mortality among newly bereaved older persons.

In the effort to learn to live without his other half, a surviving husband may try to get over the shock and to ameliorate the ensuing loneliness by moving in with one of his children, preferably a daughter. A parent does not have the same feeling of being a welcome addition to the son's house. The fact is that a parent will feel free to speak his mind with a daughter, no matter what her age, but will feel self-conscious in his contact with a daughter-in-law. The reason for this is that the daughter-in-law came into the family as an adult, while one's own daughter always remains a child to her parents.

As a rule, a widower will stay in the home of a child only temporarily and eventually branch out for himself.

If a woman loses her husband, she may for a time try to make her home with one of her children, again preferably a daughter. There she has to learn to accept the fact that she is not the mistress of her child's house. No household can tolerate two mistresses and remain peaceful for long. The present trend of aged parents living apart from their children bears out this fact. It seems that both parties prefer their independence. They want to live near each other, but not with each other. Only if the daughter or daughter-in-law follows a calling of her own that keeps her away from home during the day, and if there are small children to be taken care of, can an elderly widow find a place where she is needed and appreciated.

If a woman has remained a homemaker as long as her husband was alive, she must, after his death, not only adjust to being and living alone but also learn to manage her own affairs. Her married children frequently live far away, and it would be inconvenient for them as well as for the widow if she had to communicate with one of them for every detail in her life.

HOW NATURE HELPS

After the first shock of losing one's spouse has passed, the psychic mechanisms that come into play contribute a great deal to healing the wound and to helping the surviving mate regain equilibrium. One of the important elements of the process of mourning is the unconscious identification with the lost love object. The purpose of this mechanism is to keep the image and the memory of the deceased alive within oneself, diminishing to a considerable degree the sense of the loss as well as the subsequent isolation and deprivation. It is often quite surprising to see how far this identification can go. A widow may suddenly discover an interest in her late husband's occupation, where she previously had none, and develop a talent to a degree neither she nor her husband ever dreamed of. When she takes over the business, not infrequently she is as successful as or more so than her husband ever was. Perhaps this expectation is behind the frequent practice of installing the widow of a politician who dies during his term to serve for the remaining time —but there may be more practical (and political) motivations behind it too.

Another form of identification with the deceased is the posthumous attribution to him of things he said and did or did not say or do. These references are never derogatory or critical. On the contrary, they sometimes lead to the idealization of the deceased— to the surprise of the family and friends who knew him as he really was. This idealization is rooted—at least in part—in unconscious guilt feelings toward the deceased concerning grievances that occurred over the course of years and were never aired or resolved. In any human relationship there are unavoidable incidents one wishes had never taken place, and after the death of the mate there is no further opportunity to make amends. It is here that the family can be of great help: understanding and kindness can go a long way to assist the survivor in regaining equilibrium. The family can and should encourage the widowed parent to seek out old friends and to renew old ties, people with whom he or she could relive the past as it was possible to do with the spouse. They can try to interest the old person in some activity that would give pleasure and satisfaction and restore the sense of being wanted and, perhaps, needed. Moving out of the old house is sometimes a help. In other instances, psychotherapy may be called for, in combination with chemotherapy.

A goodly number of people will find new strength to keep on living by intensifying their religious affiliations or renewing them if they had neglected them. It is in time of stress that people remember that they had a religion.

HOW MEDICINE HELPS

Prolonged diseases force many older people into a change in their usual mode of living. But here too something encouraging can be observed. Not only do people get older at a much later age than our forebears did, but modern medical discoveries have also provided remedies for just those illnesses that have made life hard for the aging person in the past. Quite a few of these prolonged or recurrent illnesses have become in part curable or controllable to such an extent as not to handicap the activities of the elderly person. To name just a few: insulin controls diabetes, various forms of arthritis can be kept in check by medication or other means of treatment, high blood pressure can be reduced to tolerable levels, various forms of treatment take care of gastric upsets, circulatory disturbances can be helped with the pacemaker or surgery. All these methods have given their recipients a new lease on life.

The last but by no means least important event demanding reorientation in the lives of the aged is retirement.

Five

RETIREMENT: FANTASY AND FACT

*F*or the last thirty years, the sixty-fifth birthday has been a day not of celebration but of fear. It is the day when most gainfully employed people are declared to be too old to continue in the jobs they have held for many years. Even though a worker has known that this day is in the offing, its arrival is a shock from which it is difficult to recover.

While the drastic consequences of retirement are well known to experts, most people are not prepared for the fundamental, and often unwelcome, changes in store for them. They will have to adjust to living on a vastly reduced income, sometimes not enough to live on—at least not on the standard they have been used to—which in turn frequently makes it necessary to move to smaller living quarters in a poorer neighborhood. It is also liable to mean separation from old friends and familiar surroundings. The drop in social standing in the community following retirement is another blow to pride and self-esteem. As one retired man put it: "Before, I was known as Mr. X. Now, I am known as the father of Mr. X., Jr." As proud as the man may be to have a successful son, having to live in the son's reflected glory instead of in the limelight himself demands considerable adjustment and resignation. Moreover, many a man has identified himself not only with his work but also with the prestige of the company he worked for, and when he loses this prop, too, another source of satisfaction and pride is lost with it.

THE ADVERSITIES OF INACTIVITY

The change from an organized and structured work week to a life of enforced idleness is a shock that weighs more heavily on the aging worker than all the other pressures resulting from retirement, unless he is properly prepared for his new mode of living. When mandatory retirement was first instituted, there was no preparation of any kind—although warning signals for the danger it threatened already existed: during the Great Depression it had been observed that the prolonged inactivity of the unemployed worker demoralized him more than his ensuing poverty. Yet at that time, the attention of the authorities was centered mainly on the younger worker, and no one was really concerned with the repercussions involuntary and permanent idleness would call forth in the retiree. Didn't he get his Social Security payment? What else did he expect? The only excuse one can offer for this seeming callousness is that the interaction of external and internal stress in the lives of human beings was not well enough understood to stimulate measures to prevent these dangers or even ameliorate them.

Yet we all know that as much as we enjoy the weekend, when we can do as we please—especially sleep late; as much as we hate to get up in the morning to go to work during the week, free time as daily fare eventually becomes just as much a burden as rising early on a working day. To avoid the boredom that results from idleness, we resort to escapist activities. The man who has nowhere to go after he leaves the house in the morning often enough winds up at the next bar and may well become an alcoholic or a drug user. Other idlers stay at home glued to the radio or television, resenting any interruption of their programs, while still others begin to concentrate on their state of health or become depressed and sometimes end up in suicide.

Regular activity is essential in the life of every individual for the maintenance of the emotional and physical balance that safeguards our health. It was one of Freud's great contributions to give us the reason for this. He explained that no other mode of living ties the individual so firmly to the realities of life as does work, through which man becomes an integral part of society. The value of work is enhanced by the possibility it offers of expressing one's drives and instincts in most of their ramifications to a sufficient degree to maintain emotional equilibrium without giving rise to guilt feelings.* If a person is fortunate enough to follow a calling of his own choosing and to his liking, these values become even stronger. It is also a well-known fact that grief, disappointment, and other forms of emotional suffering can be best and most speedily overcome by work. If a person is deprived for any length of time of this outlet, he is apt to "take it out" on his own person, with detrimental consequences. To this class belong the escapist activities just described: feeble and useless attempts to dull one's senses and to forget one's miseries by self-damaging means.

WHEN THE DAYDREAMS
OF RETIREMENT COME TRUE

Daydreaming and escapism are common phenomena in everyone's life and have to be differentiated from planning. When a child feels stymied by parental authority, he will console himself by thinking: When I am grown up, I shall do such and such. This such and such is usually the precise thing he is forbidden at the moment.

* Sigmund Freud, *Civilization and Its Discontents*, standard ed. (London: Hogarth Press, 1930), vol. 21, pp. 108ff.

Escape into fantasy helps to make a dismal reality more tolerable, especially as long as the prospect of hope is justified. The same holds true when a hard-working middle-aged man or woman dreams about early retirement. It is quite natural to hope for a better future when the present becomes too difficult to bear and when the monotony of life takes away the joy of living. As the years go by, and the date set for the planned retirement comes closer, however, most of these dreamers begin to reconsider and postpone as long as they can the date that was supposed to bring them freedom.

The man and the woman who retire without definite and realistic plans for the future are likely to suffer from the consequences of their unwillingness to face this turn in their lives squarely. Often hopes and dreams formulated in youth cannot easily be carried out in old age. A great many people defer to their retirement years the fulfillment of the ambitions they had when they were young and that they could not satisfy at that time; when one has to earn a living, it is not always possible to write "the great American novel" at the same time or produce paintings better than Picasso's or create sculptures better than Michelangelo's. Also, the condition of the body and the general state of health at the time of retirement were usually not taken into consideration originally. No matter what the plans, neither the body nor the mind of an older person is elastic enough to meet all the demands a young person's fantasy can dream up.

Most people whose life has been tied to a rigid routine may dream of traveling. But even in the healthy aged, if the program is too rich, mental and physical fatigue will mar the pleasure. Then the wish to stay in one place becomes paramount, because the body of an aging person needs rest, relaxation, and regulated living—none of which can be obtained when one keeps moving from place to place.

Others dream of reading all the books they did not have

time to get to, seeing all the museums they could not visit before, playing on all the golf courses around the world, eating all the dishes that various countries specialize in, sailing oceans, climbing mountains or whatever else a frustrated person visualizes in his spare time. They may even attempt to follow through for a time, but every dream pales eventually if it becomes daily fare.

BACKLASH OF COMPULSORY RETIREMENT

The indiscriminate application to every worker of compulsory retirement at sixty-five caused resentment in the one who felt that he was not old enough to be sent out to pasture. It also proved to be a disadvantage to a great many employers. They began to feel the loss of the seasoned older worker's experience, as well as his greater stability. They came to recognize that an older worker was, after all, more valuable in many instances than a younger one. The older ones were not so expendable as they were assumed to be in our youth-oriented society.

Unquestionably the younger worker is more efficient than the older where speed is of the essence. The slower movements of the older man do not cope well under pressure of time and can cause confusion and errors. Yet when jobs demand special accuracy and patience, the older worker outstrips the younger one by far. In addition, the older worker has a better attendance record than the younger one; through his training and years on the job, he has know-how that the younger one cannot yet have and often does not take the trouble to acquire.

ALTERNATIVES TO RETIREMENT AT SIXTY-FIVE

The rule of mandatory retirement at sixty-five, until recently rigidly adhered to, is no longer strictly followed. In some industries, this compromise has been arrived at: when a worker is of special value to his employer, he is discharged at sixty-five and rehired on a free-lance basis. Other companies have raised the retirement age to sixty-eight in specific instances. In several fields, retirement is later: professionals in academic jobs need not retire until they are sixty-eight, and teachers in the primary and secondary schools may continue their work until seventy.

Some government employees are prepared for retirement over a five-year period: the first year, they are given one month's vacation; the second year two; the third year three; and so on to the day they must retire. During these long periods of free time, they have the opportunity to acquire new interests and skills that can fill the period of prolonged leisure that lies ahead of them.

Various plans are also being tried in which the workload and the time spent on the job are tapered off, with corresponding reduction in pay, as is only fair.* Other alternatives are to shift the worker to lighter jobs than before, to make use of qualification tests, or to rely on the worker's own determination of his job future. The last of these seems questionable, since, as Harold Geist asserts, "unfortunately most human beings are prone to underestimate their own feelings and refuse to recognize the decline of their abilities."

Several large companies ease mandatory retirement for some of their executives in this way: After the fateful day—his sixtieth birthday—has arrived, the now retired officer goes on a well-earned vacation and returns afterward to work for a time on "special" jobs for his former employers. He is often sent abroad or to other parts of the country, like an elder statesman on a delicate mission. During the months of this new activity, he has time to make new contacts and lay the groundwork for some new connection in which his old skills can be utilized.

A recent government ruling provides an additional advantage

---

* Harold D. Geist, *The Psychological Aspects of Retirement* (Springfield, Ill.: C. C. Thomas, 1968).

to the delayed-retirement worker; since Social Security premiums have to be paid whenever a worker receives wages, the amount of the benefit he receives when he finally retires is that much larger.

The above are simply examples taken at random of the range of methods that are being applied and experimented with by industry and labor. They are a further proof that mandatory retirement is no longer so strictly applied as it used to be. The practice will become still more flexible as more experience is accumulated in this field.

These alternatives have an immeasurable advantage for the worker. Not only is his economic status protected for some time to come but his self-esteem is enhanced by the recognition that he gets from his superiors and his peers. If he is rehired to train beginning workers, he may even win appreciation from the younger generation, a feat not easily achieved in our youth-oriented society. When he finally retires, he will be prepared for it and will welcome the opportunity for rest and leisure without any feeling of defeat or of having been unjustly cast aside too soon.

RETIREMENT BEFORE SIXTY-FIVE

The weakening of the relentless insistence on retirement at sixty-five has been extended in the other direction too. At first, it was women workers who were allowed to retire at sixty-two, with a 20-per-cent cut in their retirement payment. Now, men workers have the same option. Some large companies have lowered the retirement age for their executives to sixty. Others, such as General Motors, inform them when they become fifty-five whether or not they have a chance for further advancement. In case the employee does not, he has the choice of staying until he reaches retirement age or leaving before, while he is young enough to embark on a new career.

For executives who choose early retirement, there are quite

a few organizations across the country designed to provide fellow-ship, to renew old friendships, and to form new ones.* Information can be found in the section on "Organizations" in Appendix A.

Automation is constantly reducing the number of workers needed to maintain production. But in many industries, seniority rights prevent the discharge of older workers before their retirement age. In some instances, a compromise is reached by which the company pays a premium for every year the older worker retires before his sixty-fifth birthday. Once he reaches sixty-five, his regular Social Security payments and pension benefits begin.

GRADUAL RETIREMENT

The self-employed are in a somewhat different situation. There is no age at which they are forced to stop or retrench their work. And once a person continues working and reaches seventy-two, he is allowed to earn as much as he is able to without forfeiting any of his Social Security benefits.

The self-employed has had the privilege of being able to regulate his working hours throughout his career, and as he gets older, he can reduce the time spent on his job in accordance with his state of health and his preferences. However, a free-lance worker's retirement is not determined by his decision alone. The work and the clients also retire him automatically. Take the example of a busy accountant who has guided his clients over a lifetime. As they get older, they retire, they die, they give up their business, they move to a different climate, and their younger successors will consult their own contemporaries. This is a hard pill to swallow; it is very similar to the torture an aging ingenue experiences when the time comes for her to switch to playing the role

---

* *Ibid.*, p. 42.

of the mother. That is why a self-employed person is often un-willing to accept his aging or even to reduce his working time gradually.

EDUCATION FOR RETIREMENT

The leaders of business and labor have come to realize the havoc wrought on retirees by the abrupt change from regular working hours to idleness, and they have begun to take measures to remedy the situation. Organizations such as the Tennessee Valley Adminis-tration and the United Steel Workers of America, for example, have worked out programs and courses that the soon-to-be-retired worker can take, together with his spouse, on company time before retirement.

Great care is taken to select speakers who are experts in their particular fields. The topics covered include: how to estimate in-come at retirement, pension income and Social Security, insurance and hospitalization, health and aging, relationships with family and friends. Group sessions and, where needed, individual consulta-tions are arranged.

Since participation in such courses is voluntary, unfortunately they are often avoided by people who are too frightened to attend them or say they are not interested. Yet it is actually they who need guidance in this respect and who would benefit from it most. Be-cause these courses go into detail about psychological mechanisms of persons faced with difficult situations in their lives, they can perhaps reach at least some of the people who have refused to face reality and finally persuade them to face the facts of their lives at this late date.

Very wisely, the spouses are included in these courses. The reason for this is that the change in the future mode of living goes beyond the job. The drop in income is rather drastic for most workers upon retiring. The income from working that a retiree may earn between sixty-five and seventy-two, together with his Social Security benefits, is usually much smaller than the full wages he earned before, and he must comply with the government's limitation on earning if he does not want to lose his Social Security payments entirely. The average worker who has supported his wife and children has probably not been able to put sufficient money aside in savings to produce interest that will substantially augment his retirement income. Although he may have a pension, he will find that not all such plans are good; some of them need thorough revision. Even if his wife has worked, the paycheck she brought home was usually applied to raise the family's standard of living or to contribute to the children's education and to take care of extra expenses, such as family vacations, helping aged relatives, and the like.

THE RETIREE'S WIFE

A working wife faces another problem when her husband retires. It is likely that she can continue working if she is somewhat younger than her husband. A typical dilemma is that of a couple I know— a man in his early sixties and his fifty-eight-year-old wife. He wants to retire at sixty-five and go to live in a warmer climate, but he cannot count on any income other than his Social Security payments; his wife has quite a few more years to go in a job with a pension as well as Social Security. At this point they have not yet made a decision.

There is another reason for including the spouse—whether or not she has a job—in the preparatory courses and later in the decision-making. Since she must share the new mode of living, she ought to be informed about the details. Her own life is changing as profoundly as his, and difficulties in her mode of living will arise, and ensuing conflicts must be resolved. Having her husband home all day sometimes interferes with the activities she entered into after the children were grown up. The problem can best be described with the saying attributed to the wife of Casey Stengel, the beloved manager of the Yankees. When her husband retired, Mrs. Stengel was reported to have said to him: "I married you for better and for worse, but not for three meals a day."

This quip is amusing and applicable in a great number of marriages where husband and wife have remained companions and have shared their lives actively. Unfortunately, there are quite a few marriages where the crisis of retirement can also precipitate a crisis in the marital relationship. When a husband retires and spends more time at home, their relationship is bound to enter another phase. Busy as they both were in their respective spheres of activity, some couples did not realize that they had almost stopped communicating with each other. They had become simply roommates, each one absorbed in his or her own interests. Now they are forced to find their way to each other on a new basis. If this readjustment fails, the emptiness may prompt the husband to look for another woman, usually a much younger one, who seems to "understand" him better than his wife. Such crises must be faced and the conflicts resolved as best they can. With forbearance, good will, and the realization that twenty-five or thirty years of living together cannot be wiped out with a divorce decree, the husband's "fling" may pass; the wife who had let herself go and had become a disheveled old woman may pay more attention to her appearance, may change her habits, and a new approach to each other may possibly be achieved. I recall just such a couple where the woman acquired the habit of wearing out her old clothes at home and paying no attention to her grooming and general appearance except when going out. Implicit in this lack of respect for the partner is the other extreme, when a woman uses the joint bedroom as a beauty parlor. As one husband put it to me: "My wife goes to bed with cold cream all over her face and curlers in her hair. How can you make love?" As long as the man was preoccupied with his job, he may have welcomed the respite from marital duties, but now, as he relaxes at home, he wants to get reacquainted with his wife as a woman. It is not only women who commit these errors; husbands share in the transgressions too. Grievances are stored up and eventually explode. These and other topics, such as the development of common interests and the sharing of hobbies, friends, and other activities, should be included in the courses in preparation for retirement, in which both—husband and wife—should participate.

One needed innovation might be the husband's willingness to lend a hand in the household chores, but this, too, will have to be agreed upon between them. Otherwise one of them will feel victimized, with subsequent resentment and discord.

THE COUPLE RETIRES

Let us consider the case of a husband, seven years his wife's senior, who had been retired for a few years, while his wife continued on her job. He was a semi-invalid and contented himself with doing most of the household chores to make things easier for his wife. He hoped that after her retirement they could do some things together, such as going on short trips, visiting relatives and old friends. When the wife did retire, she was so scared of being idle and of being at liberty all day that she undertook so much work in charity organizations that she was busy not only in the daytime, but also in the evenings. The neglected husband responded with a depression that made his chronic illness needlessly worse. He did not dare to discuss his discontent frankly with his wife, although the connection between his emotional state and the worsening of his physical condition was pointed out to him. It took quite a while for his wife, who was actually very fond of her husband, to unwind sufficiently to get used to not having to punch the time clock every morning.

In fact, there are countless stories to be told about the pleasures aging couples find in retirement. Free time and the lessening of external pressure allow them to discover each other again, to enjoy each other's company, and to develop interests in activities they can share. Among the household chores the husband usually starts to share, cooking is one that not infrequently a man may like. The time saved for both can be spent on a hobby the two are involved in and in participating in various social activities, serving in causes, seeing friends, and the like. I have been watching a couple who live in my neighborhood. The man retired about ten years ago. Husband and wife are simply inseparable. It is heartwarming to see them going out early in the morning, rain or shine, to do the marketing together. On very rare occasions, I have seen the husband go out alone. Then he explains that his wife is not feeling well. By now rather advanced in years, they have acted as one ever since I have known them.

Another group of retirees are the people who have been able to stay on the job until seventy—for instance, schoolteachers. This group has had an "innate" training for retirement, because of the long vacations the teaching profession enjoys. They, therefore, had the opportunity to acquire interests of some constancy with which they filled the time during vacation and which they can now expand for as long as they wish.

THE HUMANIZATION OF RETIREMENT

It is clear that the humanization of retirement is now well under way, after the original implacable insistence on forcing a worker out of his job at sixty-five. It is to be hoped that this new trend will persist and eventually make it possible for an older person to accept himself and his lot, and give him the means to enjoy being old and able to make the best of his last years.

Encouraging signs are efforts by companies to preserve not only retirees' economic status but also their psychological props. Some companies are developing more meaningful pension plans, so that the worker can accumulate reserves for retirement. Steps are also being taken to preserve his feeling of belonging so that he may retain his self-esteem by continuing to identify with his former company. The retired worker is included in company social affairs; he receives the house organ. If he had worked for a railroad, he continues to have a pass for train travel after retirement. Similarly, a telephone worker has a free telephone for life. Various companies maintain other small benefits for retirees that they were permitted to enjoy during their active days at work.

The beneficial results of these improvements can already be discerned. The aging worker begins to accept retirement more easily than he did before the various fringe benefits were as well worked out as they are now—a fact that contributes greatly to his retaining self-respect and emotional well-being. Some present-day retirees may not appreciate sufficiently these attempts to rectify the grave injustices done to retiring workers in the past. A great deal of work is still to be done in this field of human relations, and older people could fruitfully fight for more improvements. We shall see in the following chapter, on the use of leisure, that fighting for a just cause is an exquisite method to recapture the zest for living.

HELP IN ORGANIZING LIFE IN RETIREMENT

Various senior citizens' organizations, such as the American Association of Retired People, as well as industry, labor, and government agencies, have joined forces not only to prepare the retiree for his new status but also to give him useful hints on how to organize his new life. For those who either must work to augment their income, or want to, they furnish a list of suitable jobs. There are companies all around the country that employ only retired workers; there are schools with very high scholastic standards that employ only retired teachers. Any retiree who is looking for work can obtain the addresses of these establishments and of other places that specialize in employing part-time workers. The Administration on Aging of the Department of Health, Education, and Welfare prepares a fact sheet from time to time to inform the aged about the kinds of jobs that are available to them. All of them pay at least the prevailing minimum wage; some pay a little more as well as transportation and other benefits.

Another possibility is the program called Green Thumb, initiated by the National Farmers Union, which operates in seventeen states. Employees work three days a week on conservation and community improvement, providing plants and shrubs for school yards and other public buildings. Other programs offer jobs for retired teachers aiding disadvantaged children; there are openings for library assistants and many similar opportunities.

In addition, several social agencies maintain sheltered workshops for the aged. Not only do they earn a little money, but they also have an opportunity to get out of their hall bedrooms and work in well-lighted, well-kept surroundings in the company of contemporaries and supervisors with a social-service background. A further plus is that they may receive medical attention.

Older people themselves are resourceful in finding part-time jobs. In a local newspaper, I read an advertisement in which two women offered to share one job. They made it easy for their prospective employers and used their ingenuity to achieve their end.

As the age of sixty-five becomes less of a threat and the conditions of retirement become more humane, it is to be hoped that retirement will not be feared but will become something to look forward to as a reward for a lifetime of hard work.

Six

THE USE OF LEISURE TIME

*T*hrough retirement people acquire a prized possession whose value can never be fully appreciated. This possession is: TIME. Without doubt, the way in which an older person spends this priceless gift determines the success or failure of his later years. Retirement is the only period in our lives in which we can spend our time exactly as we wish—or almost exactly as we wish, since there are two possible obstacles that may limit our freedom to do so.

Naturally, one's state of health in later years plays an important part in determining one's use of time. But unless a person is completely incapacitated, he still has some freedom of choice. The second obstacle is the possibility of a job. Some retirees work because they want to continue what they had been doing; therefore, they do not fall within the limitations just mentioned. Some of these people work because they have obligations toward children who are not yet able to look after themselves or because they have relatives to whose support they contribute. Still others work in order to augment their retirement income, even if their only obligation is to themselves and their spouses.

It cannot be stated emphatically enough that economic security is indispensable for the peace of mind of any elderly person; Social Security income provides for the bare necessities of life and Medicare for the maintenance of physical health. Yet a little money above the absolute minimum for survival is needed to provide some recreation and to enable the oldster to have an occasional splurge without having to deprive himself of food or other necessities.

If you have to work, federal and state agencies dealing with the aged will provide information about the kinds of work obtainable for older workers and how these jobs can be located. If you want suggestions and instructions on how to spend leisure time, you can get that information from government agencies working in conjunction with industry and labor. The present-day aged, the men and women in their seventies and beyond, had little opportunity to become acquainted with any leisure activities when they were young because of the long working hours that prevailed at that time. A substantial reason for the dread caused among this age group when mandatory retirement was first instituted was the lack of information about what one can do with free time. As working hours were shortened, this dread diminished gradually in proportion to the growing experience in relaxation and play. It also made acceptance of compulsory retirement easier.

DIVERSIONS—THEIR VIRTUES AND LIMITATIONS

The simplest way to use free time is to engage in diversions. Their allure, however, is, as a rule, short-lived, because they serve the moment only, and every amusement runs the risk of becoming stale when repeated too often or for too long. By no means does this statement imply that diversions are not useful or not needed; all I want to point out is that they do not serve as permanent fare.

There are two kinds of diversions: those that involve the company of other people, and those that can be pursued either alone or with others. Both kinds have their functions and usefulness. In fact, each is equally important, in its own way. Man needs the company of other human beings, and he needs activity as well. The psychological importance of work has its parallel in play and leisure. Yet man also needs to spend time alone, to be by himself. He has to have time for reflection, for thinking and planning, for making decisions without outside interference.

Especially in later years, when the circle of close friends diminishes, it is necessary for every older person to learn to spend time by himself, to occupy himself without other people, because companionship is no longer so easily available as it used to be. The healthiest way to spend one's time is a mixture of both: with others and with oneself. Either of these two kinds of modes of living, if it were the only one to which you were exposed, would be equally damaging to mental equilibrium. Everybody readily understands that to live in solitude for a long period is bad. The need for privacy is not so readily understood. It is, for instance, one of the complaints of old people living in nursing homes, where they usually have a roommate, that what they miss most from their former life is privacy.

It may surprise the reader that I do not include complete inactivity as a suitable form of relaxation. Quite a few people will tell you that when they retire, all they want to do is sit and do nothing. The person who has such ideas has usually had a very hard life in which he had to do very heavy work that kept him on his feet all day. It is no wonder that sitting down is his dream of freedom to do as he pleases. Yet even if he does carry out this dream, he would sit on a bench and watch the world go by, and not, as a rule, sit in his room, isolated from the life around him. And after he has rested enough, he would gradually begin to participate again actively in social life.

All athletic activities belong in the category of social contact. While young people enjoy their athletic activities most when the competitive element is the motivating force, the older person should continue his favorite sport, but should eliminate the component of competition. We have seen in other connections that speed and age do not go well together. Compromises are needed and are made by sensible oldsters. I recently heard a lady in her seventies boast that she had been able to hold her own in a nine-hole golf tournament in which her competitors were contemporaries of hers. Compromise made this possible.

The following games and activities are deservedly popular with the older generation: bowling, shuffleboard, pitching horseshoes, playing some golf (especially putting), walking, dancing (within reason), and swimming. I have read that in the warmer climates tricycle clubs for oldsters are being established; their members make trips accompanied by a nurse, just in case a member overtaxes his or her strength. I want to stress here the need for variety in order to avoid boredom, which quickly arises in repeating any activity whose sole aim is to amuse. Nor should I omit the various spectator sports, such as football, baseball, basketball, hockey, etc.

The most common indoor diversions are games—cards, dominoes, Scrabble and other word games, bingo, checkers. Chess provides pleasure, diversion, and challenge to all ages. And many outdoor activities can be adapted to indoor use.

Solitary diversions have important functions, too. In case a person is indisposed or handicapped in his locomotion, he can while away the time by listening to radio, watching television, listening to records. He can play solitaire, try solving crossword puzzles, or put jigsaw puzzles together, and he will forget the time. There are many other kinds of puzzles demanding concentration and skill. And he can, of course, read to his heart's desire.

Reading the daily papers and magazines will help keep the older person in touch with the world, and when visitors come to see him, he can make conversation more interesting for himself and them. This latter point is important because I have often heard young people say that they do not enjoy visiting their grand-parents or other old people because "they have nothing to talk about except their ailments."

MAKING UP FOR MISSED OPPORTUNITIES

Education. Further education is an ambition cherished by more people than one might ordinarily assume. Some may, for instance, have been unable to afford to attend college because they had to earn their livelihood. One often reads a report such as this:

> . . . 13 women in their sixties, seventies and eighties received certificates of completion for courses they took under the auspices of New York City Community College. . . . [The subjects included] courses in Spanish and current events in an unusual educational program for the elderly through which 357 certificates have been awarded by six of the city's eight public junior colleges. . . . [One of the students, a Mrs. Goldman, added two certificates to the one she received last year for a course in Afro-American history.] The impetus for the college's involvement with elderly people was pro-vided two years ago, when members of the Borough Park Friend-ship Club in Brooklyn, many of them foreign-born, asked for a course in English "so that we can talk to our grandchildren."
> —*The New York Times*, February 16, 1972

These elderly students have no motivation other than to fulfill a dream of their youth. They did not know, nor did they really care, whether they would live long enough to get a degree. Their effort represents purely their desire to learn and to know, and winning a degree finally gives them the self-esteem they felt, justifiably or not, they had always lacked. Young people take long-term planning for granted, but it requires a great deal of guts and self-acceptance for an aged person to plan something without having a fair assurance of living out the number of years it would take to achieve his objective. *Projects of this kind are the greatest antidote against going to seed and the surest guarantee that the oldster will remain in contact with the realities of life.*

Turning a Diversion into a Hobby. People who have made plans for their retirement years have often maintained a strong interest in some hobby for many years; they will have a relatively easy time adjusting to their new life. They are ready for retirement and sometimes even hasten it so that they can devote more attention to their avocation.

Aims and projects do not have to be so ambitious as studying for a college degree or certificate in order to produce the same beneficial effect. Energies can be applied to whatever a person enjoys doing and endeavors to do better than he did up to now: playing an instrument, painting in a more serious way than before, becoming interested in community affairs, learning a foreign language, or collecting whatever strikes one's fancy.

I would like to point out that any of these activities can be practiced as a diversion or as a project—but the difference is substantial. A great many people collected stamps when they were children. They knew nothing about the science of stamp collecting; they simply accumulated as many as possible and boasted about the number they acquired. If collecting remains a diversion on this level, it will soon give way to another. If, however, the collector— of any age—begins to become seriously interested in stamps, their history, their origin, and the like, his pride in his collection will undergo a profound change. It will shift from pride in quantity to pride in quality. Once this point is reached, a lifelong hobby has been established. Should our collector retire, he will have at hand something to occupy his time, his mind—and his money, since any collector is kept busy improving the special quality of his collection by trading, exchanging, discarding examples of lesser interest, and obtaining more valuable ones.

This shift of accent from quantity to quality changes a diversion into a hobby; it becomes an enduring interest, much more gratifying than any diversion can be, and more absorbing, not only in depth but also in width. There are many ramifications connected with a hobby that are as engrossing as the hobby itself. By learning more about the nature and origin of one's pet activity, one gets in touch with people of similar inclinations, learns of related subjects—in short, finds one's interests expanding endlessly.

Interest in the Arts.   Some people set themselves a specific project that occupies a great deal of time and affords profound gratification. A highly respected psychologist I know decided after his mandatory retirement at sixty-eight to devote his time to learning to play a Mozart sonata to his satisfaction. This may sound like a rather modest undertaking, but in fact, because this man has always pursued demanding standards, it entails learning and practicing forever. He will have to spend many hours a day for this purpose, he will have to attend concerts and watch the way in which other artists perform. A lifelong occupation is expressed in this understatement.

After they retire, other people who are less ambitious will rediscover their interest in music and will again take up the instrument they used to enjoy playing in their youth. Quite a few amateurs get together and play chamber music; others join a larger and less demanding group playing in an orchestra for the enjoyment of themselves and their friends.

Improving one's game of chess or bridge or something along this line has a similarly stimulating effect. Some people become experts in their hobby, become so involved in it that they may start a new career. I remember a middle-aged businessman who was an amateur collector of a particular kind of glass. Through his own research he became so knowledgeable in this field that as the years went by, he became a recognized authority. People from all parts of the country—even a museum curator—asked his opinion in doubtful cases. He took great pride in meeting famous people and making new friends through his hobby. Had he tried to become a professional art expert or art dealer—as many collectors eventually do—he would undoubtedly have been very successful.

Many people continue their intellectual or artistic interests after they reach retirement age but not in the direction they followed while they were actively employed. They want to widen their horizon beyond the bounds of their former calling. To satisfy this desire, an organization of a special kind was created a few years ago: The Institute of Retired Professionals, with headquarters at the New School for Social Research, in New York City.

The institute's members consist of former professionals and executives. There is no paid staff; everything connected with the organizing and running of the institute is done by the members themselves, who are not paid. Membership is limited, and there is a very long waiting list. Members may attend classes, teach classes, lead discussion groups, do clerical work—according to their preference. A recent program listed forty-four different activities: in the arts and sciences, the physical field, excursions to sites of natural and historical interest. Undertakings of this kind, perhaps on a less ambitious scale, exist all over the country in one form or another.

CONTINUING TO WORK

I believe that the concept of leisure should also include continuing to be active in the field of one's accustomed activity well beyond the average retirement age. I am aware that parts of the definition of leisure are: "not occupied or engaged," and also: "to be permitted free, unoccupied time during which one may indulge in rest, recreation, etc." (*Webster's New World Dictionary*). However, there are people who identify with their work to such an extent that the economic aspect has become quite unimportant, while the work itself has become so much a part of their existence that life without it would become entirely meaningless. As a matter of fact, quite a few eminent professional people have continued to work without pay in their customary activity after they retired from their jobs. There is not one institution of higher learning that does not have some such people on its staff. And a great many of them make valuable contributions in their field, working as consultants, teachers, and the like. Of course, it requires tact to make such a relationship a success. They have realized that they now must take second place and should not offer advice or counsel unless asked. But it can be done, and they are in most cases welcomed and respected.

Activity of this kind is common among lawyers and judges. After having retired from the exacting demands of daily practice or of the courtroom, they welcome the opportunity to teach at law schools and to act as consultants in difficult legal situations. A few years ago James M. Roche retired as president of General Motors and accepted a position as teacher of law and a member of the boards of trustees of Holy Cross College and Tuskegee Institute. Other retired business executives join organizations such as SCORE (Service Corps for Retired Executives), through which they can provide advice to managers of smaller businesses on improving their efficiency and profits.

I know of a very successful businessman who after his retirement became the unsalaried treasurer of an old people's home. On the other hand, a banker who did not want to have anything to do with finances after his retirement became a very skillful cabinet-maker. He relaxed from strenuous mental activity by using his hands.

Artists, like writers, painters, musicians, and sculptors, are free to follow their passionately loved work for as long as they are physically and mentally able to do so. It is almost like carrying coals to Newcastle to try to enumerate the artistic giants whose careers lasted well beyond the venerable threescore years and ten. Grandma Moses and Edward Steichen, both of whom died at a very ripe age, made history in their respective fields. Grandma Moses brought "primitive" art to unparalleled popularity, while Steichen was one of the pioneers who developed photography into an art form. The cellist Pablo Casals and the painter Pablo Picasso were both active in their art past the age of ninety. Elder statesmen, such as Winston Churchill and Konrad Adenauer, lived long and useful lives, as did Bernard Baruch, whose office was a park bench in Washington. Thomas Edison, the inventive genius, and Judge Oliver Wendell Holmes lived and worked well into their eighties. Many of us oldsters would love to do likewise.

SECOND CAREERS

One does not have to be a genius in order to be able to blossom out late in life with talents one had no idea he possessed. As I was gathering the material for this chapter, I received an invitation to an exhibition of paintings by an acquaintance of mine. Already pushing eighty-eight, she was having her twelfth one-man show. But what is even more remarkable is the fact that the artist did not take a brush in hand until she was sixty-nine. She was a housewife and mother who came from a very cultured background but had no specific training or interests. In time, her children married, and when she was sixty-four, her husband died. Five years later, she started to play around with brush and colors. What began as a hobby became a life interest.

After reaching retirement age, a scientist often retains a place in the laboratory or continues his research in an office of his own and is available when his experience is needed.

Other scientists leave their laboratories on retirement and devote themselves to seemingly insignificant hobbies. But sometimes, in the end, it is through these that they make a much greater contribution to scientific knowledge and to mankind than they did in their original specialty. In 1953, the scientific community was startled by the unraveling of the age-old mystery of the whys and wherefores of the travels of the salmon all the way from the Pacific Ocean up the rivers to their Alaskan spawning grounds— and their subsequent swift deterioration and death. The sleuth responsible for these long-sought explanations was Dr. O. H. Robertson, who, until the age limit forced him to retire in 1949, had been a very famous microbiologist, as well as a well-loved teacher. He also had a hobby—fishing—and after he had to leave his academic position, he concentrated on the mystery of the salmon. He traveled with the fish, studied all he could, and finally found the answers. Although he has a distinguished reputation as a microbiologist, Dr. Robertson is better remembered and more highly esteemed for having solved the riddle of the salmon's life and death.

Two of my medical colleagues also chose rather unusual second careers. Dr. George Brewer, who was head of the department of surgery at Mount Sinai Hospital in New York, retired in 1928. He then renewed his long-standing interest in anthropology and eventually became research associate in somatic anthropology at the Museum of Natural History in New York.

The other, Dr. Ralph Colp, was later also head of the department of surgery at Mount Sinai. But he stated that he was a surgeon for only ten months of the year and an archaeologist for the other two. He retired from the hospital in 1956 and from private practice in 1963, when he was seventy. Since then, he has become a full-time archaeologist and continues to participate actively in field trips to remote sites.

As we have now seen, there are a great many people who were not at a loss about what to do with their leisure years. Usually they have had a hobby that was almost as important to them as their profession or whatever else they made their living by. What we can learn from the course of their lives after they retired from their original calling is that they came well prepared for the future use of their leisure time. George Lawton, one of the very respected pioneers in the study of the aged, remarked on more than one occasion that a person should not retire *from* unless he knew where to retire *to*. In the mid-1940s, this was a novel and daring statement because relatively few people at the time were affected by the rule of mandatory retirement. We also learn from these people that in general the broader the basis of their education, the easier it was for them to select their new calling and make a success of it.

Since you are new in the pursuit of the new interest, there is no question of competition; your only aim is to become more familiar with your new subject, irrespective of the glory you may or may not acquire.

It is not, however, given to everybody to excel in his retirement activities, nor do most people wish to do so. As a rule, an older person wants to live out the last portion of his life in fairly good health, in peace, with a group of friends and members of his family, without economic pressure—and to *be* somebody. Every one of us has a different concept of what the *be* looks like and should look like.

Ambition is not the central motivation of a well-adjusted oldster, but to be needed is central, and, for most of us, the desire to pull one's own weight is all but indispensable. There are various ways in which these aims can be achieved. Every aged person who is in relatively good shape, and has accepted the fact that time is running out, has a considerable variety of activities at his disposal that would satisfy this need to be needed and give him a feeling of self-value. So long as this self-acceptance has not yet been reached, the old person, in spite of the many choices available, will complain about boredom—because he expects to be entertained by life instead of using his own initiative.

VOLUNTEER WORK

While a great many retired people continue in paying jobs in their accustomed field, others continue on a voluntary basis. A man in his seventies who had headed a successful business designing and installing kitchens and bathrooms told me what he was doing with his free time since retirement. A friend had introduced him to an agency that specializes in the rehabilitation of physically handicapped people. He began to design and organize kitchens to be used specifically by people who are confined to wheelchairs. As he explained, the sink is lowered to the level at which a person in a wheelchair can use it as comfortably as another person does while standing. However, a standard faucet, located in its usual place in the middle of the sink, is beyond the reach of a person seated in a wheelchair at the edge of the sink. So he places the faucet at the edge so that the wheelchair can be pulled close enough for the sink to be used with ease. These are only illustrations of the various adjustments he has made in kitchens, bathrooms, and elsewhere in houses. In this way, he has helped to make the handicapped person free of the need for assistance from other people, which does much to restore the feeling of being independent. And he has also given new meaning to his own life.

Other retired people use the knowledge they have acquired in their work, such as bookkeeping, typing, library service, or other occupations, in a variety of ways. They do not have to undertake work on a major scale; a little bit helps at any time. There are numerous activities from which anyone, but especially an older person, can derive a great deal of satisfaction, if he has the proper attitude toward himself and his role in life. As long as he accepts himself, and knows and is proud of his worth, he can pursue any activity, any job, paid or unpaid, that needs to be done, especially if no one else is around to do it. Many jobs do not demand special training or eight hours' work per day. Oldsters who are fairly mobile and can still add two and two without making a mistake can fill a job for a few hours a day, be kept busy, and, if necessary, earn a little spending money to boot. If a person is financially able to forgo payment, his contribution becomes that much more valuable.

One of the people who has my unlimited respect is a woman who is nearly ninety and is still spry and healthy. An actress in her youth, she later became a speech teacher, and still later made a modest living by teaching English to foreigners in the public-school system (this is one of the few working possibilities that still has no age limit). The influx of foreign-born pupils, however, diminished in the course of time because a great many immigrants now arrive in this country with a fairly good knowledge of our language. When she was eighty-eight, her job was abolished. Far from being discouraged, although a little pressed for funds, she pursued what she had always liked and knew best: speech and language. Aware that contemporaries of hers had developed difficulties reading and writing because of dwindling eyesight, she visits them regularly, writes letters for them, and reads their mail to them. She also goes with them when they have to do marketing or shopping. Through her labors of love, these people retain contact with the world around them, and she helps them to retain their emotional equilibrium.

In these careers that were begun after retirement, there are certain similarities in spite of the diversity of the specialties themselves. First, the new center of interest was actually a hobby that had been pursued alongside the actual profession. Since this outside interest was retained, there must have been equally valid reasons that the given calling was chosen for a lifework. I think I would not be very wrong in assuming that economic or prestige factors played a part in the decision. If with retirement the economic future has become secure, the avocation can become a vocation. That was probably the case with the microbiologist who enjoyed fishing or the surgeon who became a full-time archaeologist or the lawyers or businessmen who became teachers.

One striking example of a second career is that chosen by an engineer who was employed for many years by Mount Sinai Hospital. He recently attended one of the seminars arranged by the personnel department to prepare elderly employees for retirement and revealed that he planned to enter the ministry upon his retirement. In his youth, having had no funds available, he would have had to work his way through school. He decided instead to concentrate on making a living. Now that his financial worries are over, he can follow his real inclination.

These seminars at Mount Sinai were initiated by Mrs. Jean Safirstein, for whom this is her third career. Trained as a social worker, she took her master's degree in social science twenty years later. She then became executive assistant to the director of the department of psychiatry at Mount Sinai, a job she filled admirably for a number of years. When she was sixty-four, she decided to retire from that position and work only part time. It was then that she began her present career: she organized the Retirement Consultation Service for the employees of Mount Sinai and continues to conduct it to the great acclaim of her superiors and clients. These seminars cover a variety of topics of particular interest to pre-retirees. I, for example, had the privilege of participating in one, speaking on the use of leisure time.

These second careers may enhance the personal pleasure of the retiree, yet there is another element that needs to be pointed out and for which we all ought to be grateful. Every one of the people has contributed or is contributing a great deal to the common knowledge. And intentionally or not, these people serve to stimulate the younger generation to hold on to the ideals of their youth, in the hope that they, too, may sooner or later have a chance to fulfill the seemingly unrealistic expectations of their early youth—some of what I have termed pipe dreams. Maybe we of the older generation who have had the privilege of carrying out our ideals want to counteract the threat of the growing mechanization of our day-to-day living and to preserve some of the personal, human aspects in our lives, which seem to be being swallowed up by the computer.

HELPING OTHERS—AND YOURSELF

Another way of being active and useful at the same time is to work—or, better, fight—for a worthwhile cause. And there is no more worthy cause for the aged than their own. I always wonder why old people do not make themselves heard more loudly and more strongly than they do. There are, of course, many explanations for the reticence of the aged, and one of the strongest reasons is their general discouragement and apathy, which make them expect things to be done for them instead of doing them themselves. They are also afraid of being rebuffed when making demands of any kind. In short, they are afraid of "making waves," which might make things worse than they are now. One very old man explained it when speaking of his children: "I don't want them to have the feeling they *must* come and visit with me; I want them to come because they *want* to." If the old person is belligerent, the children—that is, society—will not want to have any dealings with him.

This idea may have its value in personal and family relationships, but as far as the cause of the aged is concerned, the silent submission has lasted too long, and it is time the issues were brought into the open and frankly discussed.

A COUNCIL OF ELDERS?

It has been advocated in many quarters that the aged should take a more active part in community affairs. They have the time to devote to the common good, and they have experience accumulated over many years. The aged have played this role since ancient times, and our language bears out their function by calling the municipal authorities "city fathers." The wisdom of the elders of the tribe or city-state, men or women, was held in high esteem, and their advice prevailed over the impetuosity of the younger generation. They functioned as historians and keepers of whatever knowledge the tribe possessed in politics, strategies of warfare, magic, healing, and religious practices. Today these duties are more efficiently handled by means of our modern methods of communication, which easily keep the collective memory up to date and verified by accurate records—rather than by memory, which changes as time passes. Our medical knowledge of the process of aging and the tempo of our technical advances make man, with rare exceptions, obsolete for these decision-making jobs before he realizes it. To turn the management of community affairs entirely over to the aged would not be as helpful as it was at the beginning of our civilization, or even as it was when the Founding Fathers wrote our Constitution. Today's function of leadership in any community has become rather complex and needs more flexibility than a council of elders in the old style could provide. However, there are a great many jobs in any commonwealth where older people can be of substantial assistance, where integrity and trust are needed; they can do valuable work as assistants, watchdogs, and counselors.

I have left one group of leisure activities out of this chapter, although it is my belief that it offers the most important and most gratifying use of leisure time for the vast majority of the aged, yet it is the least well known. It is the volunteer work done by ordinary citizens, people who have only limited means to live on and no spectacular talent or scientific inclination. And yet their contributions rank among the most needed and most appreciated activities of their age group. In day centers for the aged, or alone, or working with a few friends in their neighborhood, they spend considerable time every day in mutual aid. Their work deserves the highest respect and is of paramount importance in the lives of the aged. It is for this reason that I have decided to devote a separate chapter to their activities.

Seven

VOLUNTEER WORK: A TWO-WAY STREET

*T*he skill, knowledge, and experience that are allowed to lie fallow because of involuntary retirement represent a priceless asset within the commonwealth of any nation. The leaders of philanthropic and religious organizations have been aware of this fact for a long time. It is worth noting that the success of philanthropic organizations is made possible not only by the direct financial contributions of donors but also by the fact that a great many very important jobs are filled by people who could command high pay for this work if they used their talents commercially. Some of them have even made new careers by taking over the management of these organizations after they retired from their own work. Without the interest and active participation of these philanthropists, the accomplishments of charitable organizations would be much less varied, significant, and beneficial than they are.

Yet there is a group of men and women who in their own way contribute at least as much through service to their needy neighbors as the men and women who contribute large sums of money. It is to this army that I want to pay tribute by reciting their accomplishments, because the vast majority of these workers and almost all the recipients of their deeds are to be found among the retired population. It is the poor and the old, such as a great

85

many of us, who help those who are still poorer and still older. These are the thousands of volunteers who give their time and their services to settlement houses, day centers for the aged, and hospitals, or to lonely people who have no one and do not belong to any organization.

The following description of their activities and the services they perform is intended to suggest a few possibilities to anyone who is interested in becoming a volunteer. There are almost unlimited alternatives for a would-be volunteer, and anyone who is willing to lend a hand will be welcomed.

WORK IN A DAY CENTER

If you visit a large day center, you will experience one overwhelming impression: you cannot distinguish which are the members and which are the volunteers. The volunteers may be a little younger and come there only once or twice a week for a few hours, while the members spend almost all their days there. But in their involvement there is little difference.

The volunteers supervise the various activities and teach painting, ceramics, sewing, knitting, and other handicrafts. They accompany the members on their outings to museums, exhibitions, and concerts, for which they secure free tickets. They assist in getting out the monthly "magazine," which consists entirely of contributions from members; they make a fourth at a bridge game, when needed, organize fashion shows of clothes of days gone by—the prize possessions of the members and reminders of better days.

If one of the members has been missing for a day or two, this fact is reported to the director and a member is sent around to see what has caused the absence. If the member is sick and needs to be hospitalized, that is arranged. Members, now turned volunteers, regularly visit sick members at home or in the hospital. They also visit sick people, especially children, whom they do not know. In a hospital, they help with the feeding of the patients, do errands, write letters, make telephone calls, and perform other labors of love. The hospital authorities are very pleased to have this assistance. If one of the center's members dies, a delegation of contemporaries attends the funeral.

Meals on wheels are delivered to the homebound by men volunteers using their own cars. Since they are old themselves, and must avoid straining their hearts, they are accompanied by an attendant, who carries the heavy containers of food up the stairs.

The objective of these day centers is to get the old ones out of their furnished rooms—where possible—and to provide them with company and decent food. In most centers, a hearty hot meal is served in the middle of the day for a nominal price; other centers serve sandwiches and coffee at lunchtime.

Each month, a joint birthday party is held for all the members who were born during that month, and birthday greetings are mailed for their individual birthdays. This gesture helps to diminish the feeling of loneliness that arises when a birthday is completely forgotten.

There are also afternoon Thanksgiving and New Year parties at the centers, where grandchildren of the volunteers serve as waiters and waitresses. This is a good way for teen-agers to begin to become acquainted with old age outside their own family; at the same time, it satisfies the intense desire of most aged to have some personal contact with children and young people.

All these activities are designed to keep the oldster in touch with the world and protect him at the same time.

Not all day centers for the aged have a full week's schedule. Some are open only half days, some only once or twice a week. The hours depend on the amount of money they can raise and the number of volunteers they can muster. Centers are distributed throughout the large cities, and any would-be volunteer can usually find one to work for within walking distance. In most small cities and towns, similar facilities are usually sponsored by religious organizations.

REWARDS TO THE VOLUNTEER

The various services performed by the volunteers give them the satisfaction of being needed and give those they help the feeling of being wanted. At the time that a middle-aged man or woman is ready to become a volunteer, his or her professional, business, or household duties are being greatly reduced, and the time spent in serving those in need renews the feeling of accomplishment. If the volunteer is young, it offers one more chance to get acquainted with older people as individuals rather than as a group. This experience may make it easier for the youthful volunteer to accept old age in time to come.

I should like to use a technical term here without intending it to be derogatory in any way; that is, doing volunteer work is an exquisite form of "occupational therapy," without actually being a patient.

It is not easy to recruit volunteers to work with old people. While middle-aged female volunteers are willing to work with sick children, they shy away from the aged. As an excuse, they mention a sick relative they must look after, and explain that they do not want to be involved with still more sickness in old people. Actually, it is their own attitude toward aging that is the cause of this reluctance. Introductory courses for volunteers would be most helpful, to them as well as to the cause they might decide to serve.

ONE-TO-ONE SERVICES

Among volunteer organizations, there is a large variety, offering numerous fields of activity to choose from. Those I am describing are for the most part located in New York City, the largest of the metropolises, where it is most likely that a person can disappear without ever being found. The larger organizations, however, are usually nationwide, and branches are located in most communities. In smaller towns, the people in need are usually known to the inhabitants or local authorities, and assistance there is more personal and easier to come by than in a large city.

To illustrate the diversity of volunteer activities, I will cite examples of each of the three main kinds of sponsors of volunteer activities.

The Lenox Hill Neighborhood Association is a nondenominational local agency serving people in the vicinity of all ages—from childhood, through pregnancy, to old age. Very recently, it instituted a service that is intended not only to help the old but also to bridge the gap between the generations. It enlists a number of junior- and senior- high-school students living in its area—the East Seventies—to devote some of their free time to the aged. If an old person is unable to leave the house, they run errands for him, or they accompany him when he goes shopping.

The next is a religious organization called East Midtown Services to Older People. It is sponsored by the Episcopal Mission Society. This facility, which is open five afternoons a week, is staffed by volunteers who assist old people in marketing; accompany the sick to the doctor, dentist, or a clinic; and visit the sick in their homes. It also furnishes information about part-time employment, about getting reduced-fare passes (which are also good for identification at movie theaters giving discounts). It prepares the forms for rent-increase exemptions, finds sources for financial help where needed, and takes care of securing food stamps.

A short time ago, the Federal Government, through the Office of Economic Opportunity (OEO), began to conduct a door-to-door search for people in need. It organized a group called FIND (Friendless, Isolated, Needy and Disabled), whose workers are all aged. Although the government pays them small salaries for their services, they are still classified as volunteers. No special training is required, but they must have the ability "to project interest, warmth and sympathy" and must not mind climbing stairs to reach oldsters who have lost touch with the outside world.

Even nursing homes join in contributing assistance to people in need. Every morning, some of the residents at the Florence Nightingale Nursing Home who are in good physical condition are transported to the Stanley M. Isaacs Neighborhood Center, where they man the telephones for the Telephone Reassurance Program, one of the many established all over the city, in which they chat with sick and anxious citizens.

The Community Service Society, which initiated the Telephone Reassurance Program, has recently established another activity on a much larger scale. It is called Volunteers, with the subtitle RSVP (Retired Senior Volunteer Program). It was such a success that the government became interested and took over the management as well as the funding. It pays the participants for transportation and lunch. (Under certain circumstances, they may get a small remuneration.) Volunteers consist of former teachers, secretaries, bartenders, executives, salesmen, housewives—in short, people from all walks of life. They work in the Family Court and mental hospitals; they act as aides to teachers in elementary schools and serve in day-care centers for children and the aged, in museums and in libraries (where they do clerical work and help repair and rebind damaged books); they tutor children who have difficulties in schoolwork, teach English to children and adults of Hispanic origin; feed and entertain in geriatric institutions, and do countless other tasks. Anyone willing to devote a few hours a week to this work is welcome.

The ingenuity that groups and individuals develop to help others is unlimited. The magazine *Modern Maturity* reported (No. 3, 1973) on Mae Stuart, seventy-nine, who regularly runs an advertisement in newspapers inviting people to phone her and tell her which hymn they would like her to play for them on the piano. The article stated that Miss Stuart leads a very busy life.

THE SHELTERED WORKSHOP

A sheltered workshop is usually run by a philanthropic organization or in connection with a hospital. It is a place where people of any age who are temporarily handicapped can find work they are able to perform until they are well enough to return to their former calling or to be retrained for a new occupation.

Sheltered workshops for the aged have a different basis because they are, for obvious reasons, intended to fulfill not a temporary but a long-range function. They exist all over the country and are a great help to old people who need to augment their Social Security payments but may be too proud to ask for public assistance, and who are not well enough to enter the regular labor market. Generally, these workshops have a professional director and a volunteer chairman, who is the representative of the humanitarian organization that supports the workshop. Working time is limited to twenty hours a week, and since no more than four hours' work can be done in any one day, the workers travel back and forth to work in daylight and at reduced fares. Pay is based on the piecework system, so that each person can set his own pace, without undue strain on his strength. There is a couch in the rest-

room—just in case. Although the sheltered workshop does not
provide lunches, there is a very well-kept, friendly lunchroom with
a refrigerator and stove so that the workers can prepare their own
food. The newest innovation in one of these workshops is a daily
group-therapy session held before work begins.

With ingenuity, a sheltered workshop can stretch the money
it receives from its sponsoring group and at the same time benefit
its fellow groups. There is one particular shop I want to describe
because its chairman, a woman of seventy, in collaboration with a
dedicated director, has developed the workshop from a capacity
of twenty-five to a facility that provides work for about a hundred
old people. The plan devised in this workshop is an excellent
illustration. It fills the shop's needs for printed material, such as
stationery, by buying from another sheltered workshop, where the
prices are lower than in a commercial enterprise. The chairman
explains that "The quality may not be first class, but we help them,
and they help us." The ceramics that are needed in the workshop—
ashtrays, dishes to hold needles and other equipment used by the
workers—are purchased at a day center for older people where
ceramic making is part of the regular activity of its members,
who earn a little money through the sales of their products. Three
organizations are helped by the business acumen of one enthusiastic
lady past the prime of youth.

SHARING INTERESTS AND SKILLS

For people who are public-minded and interested in local or national affairs, participation in the work of, for instance, the League
of Women Voters might be rewarding. There are many similar
organizations suited to your particular political inclinations.

Churches of all denominations, councils, and social agencies
will welcome volunteers gratefully. Every hospital has a com-

mittee of volunteer workers who help out in the gift shop, the library, and with patient services, and other activities.

The richness of opportunities and the willingness of so many old and poor people to be of help are healthy indicators of the changing attitude toward the aged. I have described these possibilities and performances in detail because I want to stimulate you to make use of your hidden talents and skills in volunteer work. Almost every one of you has a personal specialty that has given you pleasure for a long time, and you could share it now with younger people. If you have a favorite recipe that used to be your "secret," sure-fire success as a hostess, you might part with it now, since you can't take it with you. You who are craftsmen can share your skills with young people and teach them not only your craft but also pride in having produced something with their own hands instead of buying it ready-made. The satisfaction you get as a teacher when you see your pupil succeed can make the difference between vegetating and enjoying living at our age.

Eight

SEXUAL ADAPTATION IN LATER LIFE

$\mathscr{N}$o differentiation has been made in this book so far between male and female. In explaining the aged to themselves, both men and women have been considered simply as people who have to face life in pretty similar fashion. However, when discussing the adaptations in the sexual sphere that are necessary in later life, we encounter great differences between the experiences of men and of women. As obvious as these differences are, there is nothing harder to get than authentic information about this phase of later life.

Recently some data about the sexual feelings and activities of aged people have been obtained through interviews and questionnaires. But however determined the investigators were to elicit reliable information, I doubt very much that these findings are representative. The main reason for my doubt is that most people, especially older ones, and most especially older women, feel embarrassed when asked about this subject. Naturally, this prevents them from disclosing their true feelings. The interrogator in his turn is embarrassed, too, especially if he is young. He feels as if he is intruding into forbidden and very delicate territory.

Even men, who are generally inclined to boast about their virility when talking to friends, are reticent in later life when asked a serious question about their sexual state. Unless the interrogator is well acquainted with the person being interviewed, the answers are usually in the negative, because the oldster thinks that is what is expected of him. He has known all his life that an old person is supposed to have little interest in sex and is not supposed to have any amorous or flirtatious emotions. What is not only permitted to a younger person but also considered natural becomes forbidden to him, and people are quick to call him a "dirty old man."

MARRIED COUPLES

Those who are least disturbed because of sexual aging are the couples who have been married to each other for quite a long time. People who were married young and stayed together have been gradually adjusting to each other sexually over the years of their marriage. As they grew older, in most instances they hardly noticed the diminution of their sexual appetites or the change in the performance. The better they got along as people, the easier it was for them to adapt to changes in their sexual relationship. They have shared so many turning points in their lives together, good ones and bad, they have supported each other if by nothing else than their mere presence or by acting as sounding boards when one of them had to let off steam. They shared the rearing of the children, their growing up, their fortunes, and also their misfortunes in life—as parents do to a much larger extent and with greater intensity than children ever do in regard to their parents. In short, there were so many reasons why the sexual drive and its expression were sometimes in the foreground, and at other times almost forgotten, that the couple did not pay much attention when they finally realized that their sexual life had gradually receded permanently into the background. As time went on, the intervals between sexual unions grew longer by unspoken mutual consent; but sexuality very seldom ceased entirely, although tenderness and physical closeness may eventually have outlived the ecstasy of the sexual act. But even very old couples do have a fairly active sex life and do not live together only as companions.

Often, looking at an old couple, one wonders what physical attraction has remained strong enough to stimulate sexual intimacy. It must be kept in mind that people who have spent a lifetime together see each other not only as they are but also retain an image of how the other looked in the early days, like a double exposure that hides to a large extent the tell-tale signs of the passage of time. In addition, they have unconsciously imitated each other's movements and bodily expressions so that in time they resemble one another like brother and sister. And if one of them becomes aware of the lessening of their sexual activity, he usually attributes it to current reasons, such as overwork, too much athletic exertion, or other circumstances that have nothing to do with getting older.

As the couple ages, new crises have to be faced in the event that one of them becomes seriously ill. When the lasting diseases that usually appear in later years manifest themselves, not only the sex life but the whole mode of living must be adapted to the new situation. For instance, cardiovascular disturbances may impede the frequency of sexual activity or surgery may change the appearance of the body or demand special attention and assistance of a delicate nature from the spouse. It is often impressive to see how matter-of-factly this care is given and how the new situation only deepens the relationship instead of upsetting it.

Where a marriage has broken up because of divorce or because of the death of a mate, the situation changes drastically. Here the gender makes the difference, as indicated earlier. While the sexual appetite remains pretty much alike for both men and women, the opportunity for expression differs sharply between them as time goes on. The male finds almost no limitations due to age in expressing and gratifying his sexual desires as long as his physical condition remains good. When people hear about a late marriage of a well-known man, most often they will smile indulgently, almost incredulously, at the old man's "whim" and courage in taking a new wife. If she is much younger than her new husband, the reaction of his friends is sometimes: "There's no fool like an old fool." If she is near his age, there will be more well-wishers, but many people will be surprised that a person past seventy, let us say, still has such "young ideas" in his head. If an older woman marries a much younger man, heads are shaken over her folly; when she marries a contemporary, the assumption is that they are seeking only companionship. That old people can still be attracted to each other and enjoy marital life like the young is almost disturbing to younger people. This reaction reflects a leftover of the taboo that forbids the child of any age to speculate on what goes on in his parents' bedroom—especially when they are past middle age, and the guilt feelings that arise if he does.

In consequence of such prejudices and inhibitions concerning the erotic inclinations of older people—and despite growing public enlightenment—a great deal of misinformation persists. The aged themselves are not any better informed. It would be regarded as unbecoming for old persons to inquire into this topic. That is why they too continue to take numerous misconceptions as gospel truth. Many older men and women could lead a much more satisfactory existence if they knew their "facts of life" and learned to assess themselves more correctly and courageously.

MEN

Some men have the habit of bragging about their sexual conquests and irresistibility to women. What they are telling is something similar to the "tall stories" fishermen like to exchange over a drink.

Unfortunately, these stories are taken literally by some of the listeners, whose shaky self-esteem is still further diminished by such unfavorable comparisons to their own accomplishments. This brings to mind the story of one of those discouraged men. He finally consulted his physician about the problem. The doctor examined his patient thoroughly and declared him to be in very good health. The patient would not believe the doctor's statement, saying: "If I'm so healthy, how come I can't do as well as my buddies?" The doctor replied: "Well, you can talk too."

However, more factual information is available about men's sexual activities than about women's. History and biography have told us a great deal about the maintenance of sexual prowess among great men throughout the ages. How much poetic license was woven into these stories is hard to guess. Victor Hugo, the great French writer of the nineteenth century, for instance, kept a diary in which he registered the dates of his sexual activities until his death at eighty-two. In *Olympio*, his biography of Hugo, André Maurois noted that, as a rule, Hugo had sexual relations twice a week with young domestics who were engaged for this purpose rather than for housework. Since they received compensation for their services, their personal responses were of no interest to their master and were not entered in his diary.

Quite a number of very well-known men have married in their sixties, or even later, and raised a new family. Most of us know of such late unions or marriages that turned out well. One who did so was my paternal grandfather. A widower, he married my grandmother when he was sixty-six and she was forty years his junior. She bore him six children, of which my father was the eldest. My grandfather died at the age of ninety-one, a year after my father got married.

As impressive as these incidents are in testifying to the men's physical health and stamina, they all fail to report some very important elements. It is quite true that these men were able to perform the sexual act itself, that they were in many instances able to sire children. Little is known, however, about the quality of their sexual activity compared to their past performances, their emotional involvement, and how much or how little their partners enjoyed the act. After all, in a permanent relationship these elements are of great importance.

Any older man reading about these and other such accomplishments may compare his own declining efficiency and draw the wrong conclusions—usually because he does not take into consideration that the sexual apparatus is subject to the same alterations due to aging as any other organ in the body. By no means does that imply that the function stops, any more than it does in other parts of the body as we get older. There are a great many men in their seventies and over who are able to function perfectly well sexually to their own and their partners' satisfaction; they are also able to impregnate a woman if she is young enough to conceive. The performance may not be as vigorous as it was decades before, it may take more time to get fully aroused, and the act itself may not create the same ecstasy as it once did. The intervals between the individual acts may become longer until many years later they stop or cannot be fully completed because of waning physical strength.

WOMEN

Neither history nor biography neglects to mention the women who preserved their beauty and youthfulness, as well as their attractiveness to men, to almost legendary ages. One of these was Cleopatra, the queen of ancient Egypt. She enchanted Julius Caesar, by whom she had a son, and lived with Marc Antony until she died at thirty-nine. Considering that in her era life expectancy was around forty years, she would have been classified as an old woman when she captivated Antony. The other most famous female lover in history is the Frenchwoman Ninon de Lenclos, a contemporary of Louis XIV and Molière. She was renowned not only for her beauty but also for her charm, her wit, and her tact. She had many lovers who feted and supported her, until she was well advanced in years. When she died, at eighty-five, she was mourned by great men of letters, one of whom had said to her a few years earlier: "You take my advice and say 'love' boldly all the time and never let the words 'old age' soil your lips."

When Frieda, the wife of D. H. Lawrence, was forty-seven, she started a flirtation with a man twelve years her junior who was married and had three children. This affair was consummated a few years later and eventually culminated in a marriage when Frieda was seventy-one years old.

I readily concede, however, that these two *grandes dames* are exceptions; it is rare that women of advanced years are able to attract men so considerably younger than themselves. For nature has not been so generous with women as with men. A woman has fewer years to look for and find the man with whom she wants to spend the rest of her life than a man has at his disposal to make his choice. Over the centuries, women have learned to take better care of themselves and of their looks and to develop their personalities, and men too have learned to appreciate values other than external appearance. Nevertheless, when a new relationship is desired in later years, the discrepancy between the sexual attractiveness of older men and older women makes it considerably more difficult for the latter to form permanent and successful unions. The government's "Population Reports" graphically show the differences in life-style resulting from this fact. (One must keep in mind that in the total aged population—I am talking of people sixty-five and over—there are considerably fewer men than women.) Recent official "Reports" show that the marriage rate for men in this age group (73.1 per cent) is more than twice as high as the rate for women (36.2 per cent). What is even more striking is that only 17.1 per cent of men in this age group are widowers, while 54.2 per cent of women sixty-five and over are widows!* In other words, more than three times as many men as women remarry in their later years after the death of their spouse. This also proves that the new wife belongs to a much younger age category than the wife who died.

The large number of unattached older women raises the question of how they come to terms with their sexual needs. In trying to get information on this subject, even a physician in consultation with a female patient meets in most cases with silence. Unlike most men, women either refuse to speak about themselves or deny that they still have feelings about sex at all. When asked to elaborate on this subject, they refuse. It is a topic that is not discussed, and it is hardly ever mentioned in the many books that deal with research about the lives and fortunes of the aged. The reasons are obvious when we consider that the cultural background of the present-day aged is closely connected with the last remnants of mid-Victorian prudishness and hypocrisy. Their mothers taught them that sex was an unspeakable nuisance, that a respectable woman did not have any sexual desires, and that her marital duties consisted of accommodating her husband. When she became a widow, the thought did not occur to her or to anyone else that she might be missing something by not having a sex partner.

THE DOUBLE STANDARD

Women's ignorance was due to the double standard, which gave most privileges to men and few to women. Since men were assumed

* *Current Population Reports*, U.S. Department of Commerce, Series P-23, no. 43, February 1973.

to be polygamous by nature, the wife had to accept her husband's escapades. The only way she could salve her pride was to pretend that this aspect of her married life was unimportant to her.

The lack of concern about female sexuality was in part due to a dearth of information and to the conspiracy of silence in regard to sexual matters. That a woman can and should be given the opportunity to reach an orgasm during sexual intercourse has been all but unknown to men, or conveniently ignored. While modern women are writing books on female orgasm, a great many men, especially of the older generation, have no conception of what a female orgasm consists of. If you ask them, they will say that they rely on what their sex partner tells them but would not be able to distinguish a fib from the truth.

The same reticence exists among older unattached women, most of whom steadfastly deny that they have any sexual desires, needs, fantasies, and activities. Only on one occasion did I hear a frank admission about sexual desires from an old woman. During one of the group discussions mentioned earlier in the book, the topic of the day was sexual activity, and the matter of the discrepancy between men's and women's chances for gratification came up. A woman well into her seventies stated: "Women want sex too, but they don't have the opportunity."

When I started these group discussions, the very first question that was put to me at the first meeting came from a very elderly but very youthfully got-up lady: "What do you think of 'straw marriages'?" Perhaps she really wanted to know, or maybe she was simply testing my mettle, but I had to confess that I had never heard this term, and with my inquiring of the participants what it meant, the discussion was well under way. (For the uninitiated, "straw marriage" means marriage in name only, marriage without sex. Up to that time, I had always heard this kind of relationship called a "white marriage.") The question alone—not to mention the ensuing discussion—proved the intense interest old people take in sexual activities as well as in marriage.

FACTS AND FALLACIES ABOUT MENOPAUSE

A profound misconception is caused by the fact that until recently the organic occurrences during menopause were not properly understood, and a great deal of ignorance still exists among a large portion of the general public. The most prevalent fallacy is the belief that once a woman stops menstruating or has her uterus removed by surgery, she no longer has any sexual feelings. As the saying goes: "She ceases to be a woman." Nothing is further from the truth.

Without going into elaborate detail on the subject, I think some explanation is needed. The sexual apparatus is very complicated; the ramifications and interactions among the ovaries, the uterus, and other hormone-producing organs are so closely connected and the psychological superstructure is so interwoven into the total personality that after the ovaries stop functioning, a realignment of the remaining hormones takes place that enables a woman to react in the same way as a female as she had before—provided she and her husband accept the fact that she remains the same person. Actually, some women enjoy their sexual activities even more after this occurs because they need no longer fear pregnancy.

As a woman reaches her seventies, her sexual apparatus is also subject to local changes, even if her feelings and desires remain active. Just as with the male, it may take her longer to respond to sexual stimulation. There is a diminution of elasticity in her vagina, leading to a degree of rigidity in the tissue, especially at the entrance. Women who continue their sexual activity with their husbands on a more or less regular basis may not even become aware of this; it becomes more noticeable when a woman has had no sexual activity over a considerable period of time. As folklore puts it: "After seven years of chastity, a woman becomes a virgin again." This point is worth noting, because if a woman does resume sexual activity after a long interruption, she may experience pain at first, and it will take a great deal of tenderness and patience from her partner to help her to overcome this hurdle.

A common sign of aging is the development of fibromas—benign tumors—around the time of menopause or even earlier. These necessitate surgery. Something similar takes place in men in their sixties when the enlargement of the prostate gland also demands surgical treatment. After this, men too retain the ability to become sexually stimulated, and most of them continue to be able to carry out the sexual act without major difficulties.*

SEXUAL SUBSTITUTES

Since time immemorial people have resorted to masturbation as a means of releasing sexual tension when no partner was available. The various religions and the moral codes of most past cultures have frowned on this practice. Parents, teachers, and the clergy punished children when they discovered them engaging in such activities, and the most dire consequences were threatened for the future mental and physical health of the child who "abused" himself or herself in that fashion. The elders thus succeeded in implanting these children with guilt feelings that lasted throughout their lives, notwithstanding later, better knowledge. There are also other powerful sources for the deep-seated guilt feeling arising in childhood masturbation. As a matter of fact, modern psychiatry

* Anyone who wants to learn more about these two occurrences is referred to an excellent book written for the layman: Isadore Rubin, *Sexual Life after Sixty* (New York: Basic Books, 1965).

knows that this feeling is caused not by masturbation as such, but by the fantasies that accompany it. To discuss this in detail goes beyond the scope of this study. Suffice it to say that a great many adults still regard self-gratification with the same horror and the same guilt feelings as they did when they were little. And if an unattached adult resorts to this "crime," he or she is not likely to divulge the "secret" readily.

Initially, there were very valid reasons for such universal condemnation of self-gratification. The Bible commanded that men and women should multiply and become as numerous as "the sands of the earth." In all early civilizations, the fathering and bearing of children was equally essential for the survival of the tribe because of high infant mortality. This reason has certainly lost its validity in the face of the present-day threat of overpopulation; moreover, most of the women who are forced to seek this kind of relief from sexual tension for any length of time are usually beyond the child-bearing age.

My efforts to get information on this delicate subject have yielded very meager results. Very few older women even admitted to me that they still had sexual desires. And they did not tell me what they were doing about it. When one or another finally owned up to the fact that she helped herself by masturbation, she did so in such a circumspect manner that one could easily see how much it had cost her to make the admission, as if it were a crime to be human. When I asked one woman of seventy, whose husband was ten years older than she and a semi-invalid, whether she still had sexual activity, she answered in a roundabout way. She blushed and said: "No, I do not, but I have my fantasies."

Another example was related to me by a colleague. This aged patient's husband was also an invalid and unable to be sexually active. At first the patient denied any interest, but a little later she reluctantly admitted that she did indeed satisfy herself.

With this, she started to leave the office, but before closing the door, she poked her head around it and added defiantly: "And I enjoy it too."*

I have encountered only one instance of a woman in her middle sixties openly admitting her desire for sexual activity. She came for consultation, bringing with her her husband, who was slightly older than she. It was her complaint that her husband had lost all interest in sex, while she, recently retired from her job, had hoped that they would now begin a new life, including more sexual contact. As it turned out, the husband was suffering from an organic disease, not yet diagnosed, that precluded his sexual activity.

Some women as well as men in their eighties and over are still interested in remarriage in the fullest sense. I was once consulted by a forty-year-old woman who had been having an affair for many years with a man who was then eighty. Although his income was meager, he had financed her professional education. She had always hoped he would finally marry her, and they seemed to be devoted to each other. She described the extent of their sexual relationship. He was able, at times, to be aroused and to perform the act to their mutual satisfaction. At other times, he was able to have an erection and enter, but did not have sufficient physical strength to finish the act.

To her great shock he informed her one day that they must part company. I asked the gentleman to come to see me. He readily explained his plight. After working for many years, he had retired on a small pension. This was before Social Security had been introduced, and the pension was not large enough to maintain his modest standard of living, especially after the young woman came into his life. So he apportioned his savings, which were modest enough, for the number of years he expected to live. Now he had

* Verbal communication, courtesy of my friend Dr. Mary Eleston.

lived longer than he had anticipated, and his savings had been used up. The only way he saw for survival was to marry a rich woman. And he knew such a woman, who was eighty-six and anxious to get married again, and he wanted to enter the hoped-for relationship clear of any obligation to his young lady.

OTHER SUBSTITUTE GRATIFICATIONS

Not all men or women without partners resort to masturbation, or they may do so only occasionally. There are quite a number of ways in which a person can, at least temporarily, ignore his sexual feelings. Some people lose themselves in causes and become so completely identified with them that they have no energy left for any other form of pleasure. Others become absorbed in a job to such a degree that it uses up all their energies. One can see their counterpart in men much younger whose wives complain that they are married to their business and not to their spouses.

Various games can become so compelling that routine human activities—including the sexual ones—are forgotten. Watching the faces of the participants around a gambling table bears out this contention. Similarly, I know a number of older women who are so devoted to playing bridge or other games that they hardly even take time out for meals. This substitute gratification of the sexual drive is not confined to females or to any specific age. Anyone who is familiar with life in a day center for the aged will have seen men coming in the minute the door opens and sitting down to their card game without budging until closing time. Serious gambling is not allowed in these places—the stakes are pennies—but the fascination with the game is as great as if they were playing for millions. The people in charge of such centers find it very hard to break up these steady games and to interest the players in more sociable activities.

Other lonely people take to drink in order to forget what human contact is like. Loneliness is by far the most painful experience and the greatest punishment to which a man or a woman can be subjected. It may lead in some instances to an exaggeration of self-love expressed in self-observation—as for instance in the state of one's health, moods, or various functions of the body, culminating in hypochondriasis. These are the people whose favorite topic of conversation is past and present illnesses and operations.

Physical contact, such as caressing, simple touching, seeing, hearing, and the other kinds of stimulation through the sense organs are essential parts of the sexual drive, and sometimes partial gratification can go a long way toward making it possible to tolerate the absence of complete sexual activity. Especially if the drive itself begins to diminish as time goes on, the presence of other people whom one knows well becomes vital. Some dote on a dog, a cat, or a pet of some other kind. This is more than mere companionship. This is a form of love.

Some older people, however, really do succeed in repressing all their conscious sexual desires and live in celibacy to the end of their days. Yet some personality traits can be discerned that prove how difficult it is to achieve the abstemious life. Old people who live that way neglect their appearance as if to defy anyone who might befriend them. They turn their longing for love into anger and hostility, become quarrelsome and intolerant; they are the first ones to condemn a younger person, or even a contemporary, for that matter, who chooses to live a freer life. No matter how strongly some old people disapprove of the sexual revolution taking place at the present time, their protests are often based on reasons other than moral outrage. If we consider how restricted a life present-day aged women were forced to lead in their youth, one can readily understand that part of this indignation is caused by pure and simple envy. How different might their lives have been if they had had only a portion of the freedom today's youth enjoy. Being old myself, I cannot help keeping my tongue in cheek when I use the word "enjoy." The present-day youngsters, in their eagerness to do what their best friend is doing, through their absolute lack of discretion and their indiscriminate acceptance of the assumption that freedom and license are synonymous, are depriving themselves of the most valuable thing in life—love. I do not know whether this train of thought fits into a book on aging, but I should not be surprised if quite a number of my contemporaries agree with me. Just to finish this excursion in my thinking: I am convinced that what is going on at the present time among young people is a temporary fad, which will pass and which may lead to a more realistic and more idealistic philosophy of life in the future.

The need for human contact and for physical proximity is at no time greater than in old age, when they serve as reassurance that there is someone who cares, and there are people for whom one cares in return. I know from personal experience that some of the old go for years without touching a human being other than by a handshake. This point was driven home to me by the story of a very old lady who, while sitting in a bus, made the acquaintance of a young woman who had a two- or three-year-old child on her lap. By some chance the child put her arms around the neck of the old lady. The old woman began to cry. She had all but forgotten how it felt when a little child caressed her. Recently the government has instituted a project in which the aged serve as foster grandparents. Much better than any words can, this move acknowledges the general need for this experience and also the beneficial effect it has on the child.

REMARRIAGE

Just as the most successful sexual adjustments between couples in later years are made by those who were compatible as people, so the most successful later marriages are based on a combination of sexual and temperamental compatibility. A woman need not be a Ninon de Lenclos to retain her attractiveness to men as the years go by. A good head on a woman's shoulders and a good education, as well as the ability to support herself or at least to contribute to the family treasury, give her a different status in the eyes of men, which substantially extends the years of her attractiveness to them. With education and work experience, women have been developing self-esteem and learning to meet men on their own ground. Far be it from me to advocate, as the modern Women's Lib adherents do, competition with men. A woman ought to complement the man of her choice and vice versa, instead of foolishly trying to outshine the mate. In the marriages that endure and the families whose children grow up into reliable personalities, there is mutual respect between the couple, and their common interests outlasted the honeymoon.

Similarly, marriages entered in later life under the same conditions have a much better chance of success and a realistic expectation of lasting, especially when the temperaments of the couple have sufficiently advanced to appreciate that compatibility and community of interests are equal in importance to sexual attractiveness.

NEW OPPORTUNITIES

The "contagion" of greater sexual freedom—without its excesses, to be sure—can be discerned by any interested observer in a day center for the aged, a senior residence, or an old people's home.

Although all the events in old age occur at a slower and less intense pace than they do in earlier years, the goings on in most of these centers for the aged are very similar to the parallel goings on in young people's singles clubs. There is the "femme fatale" of seventy, who plays her contemporary suitors one against the other, just as she did at eighteen; there are rivalries among the women for the favors of some of the men who are outstanding either because they are well preserved or because in their earlier years they were more prominent than the other men or because they have some other source of special attraction. There are women trying to get husbands, just as they did when they were younger, and there are men scouting around for a prospective wife who is supposed to have some money hidden in the cookie jar or to be a good cook. And there is a good chance for mutual satisfaction in such a search. As one woman who had just married one of her fellow day-center members explained to me: "You don't eat well unless you cook for a man."

Actually, although marriages result from the daily meetings at the centers, some of the couples live together without a marriage certificate—though often with their clergy's secret blessing. An arrangement of this kind is usually made for economic reasons. If, for example, a woman who is divorced and receives some alimony should remarry a man who has not much more than his Social Security benefits, she would forfeit her alimony, and both of them would be worse off financially than before. Another example: if a man who is already retired and receives a pension marries again, the new wife is not entitled to a widow's pension. And if a woman who has a widow's pension remarries, she will lose the income.

Some time ago, I saw a film on television of two inmates of an old people's home who had gotten married. They were both in their eighties. They seemed very happy and explained that they both enjoyed television, but the rules of the house did not allow people of different sexes to be in a room alone together. There must have been more to their decision to get married than the pleasure of watching television in company; they could have had the company of their respective roommates. But there is a difference between living with somebody and belonging to someone. In their code of ethics, it was the legality that made the difference. This story shows that loneliness exists even in crowds and that the feeling of belonging exclusively to one person comes very near to being in love with that person. Both these old people were probably too embarrassed to admit to the world their need for each other, and it was rather moving to see the reaffirmation that emotions in old age are no different from those in youth—though maybe less stormy.

The attitude of adult children toward the remarriage of elderly parents varies according to their relationship with the widowed parent, the stepparent they will acquire, and other circumstances. This topic will be discussed in detail in Chapter 10.

HOMOSEXUALS

In our time of sexual revolution, a word must be said about the way homosexuals fare in later life. Now that they are free from fear of blackmail and extortion, the young ones are sowing their oats like any other young people. But their future does not look so bright; then they will not be able to get partners in sexual activity so easily as they used to. It is in the nature of homosexuality that the relationships between partners are different from relationships based on heterosexuality. Few homosexuals—of either sex—enter a relationship on a permanent basis, which is the basis of marriage. Loyalty to each other and emotional ties are of a rather tenuous nature, and the relationships tend to be short-lived.

If the pair does settle down to some form of permanence,

many more concessions have to be made to keep them together than is the case in a heterosexual union. As time goes by, the two become roommates or business partners, or the relationship turns into that of a parent and child, but sexually they go their own ways as best they can.

Eventually, the older one has to take the back seat, and he will find it increasingly harder to get a suitable partner, even on a temporary basis. In homosexuality, each one fundamentally seeks in his partner the youth he once was. As long as both are young, this role is alternated between them. With advancing years, the older one is more and more forced to accept the parent role toward the youthful lover, a self-deception that cannot go on forever because he looks for his own youth in his partner. And since the latter seeks the same, the older one becomes in time unacceptable to the younger one, and the relationship loses much of its mutuality. This delicate situation demands more sacrifices and self-abnegations of the older of the pair than he can take in the long run. As a result, the relationship breaks up, and there is more isolation.

Once the battle has been fought out within the older one and he accepts the parent role, they can continue living together and develop a human relationship of loyalty and friendship, especially as the younger one, as time goes on, ages too.

Since every individual has one parent of the same sex and one parent of the opposite, some heterosexual tendencies are unavoidable in any homosexual person also. These tendencies have been repressed because of fear of the sexual demands made by a member of the opposite sex. In later life, the way is now open toward social companionship with members of the opposite sex. Moreover, to be on the safe side, male homosexuals usually choose the company of women older than themselves, thus providing a reservoir of escorts, friendships, and companions for unattached women who are no longer particularly interested in sexual activity or in getting married. This situation has advantages for both sides. There are so many more older women than older men, and involuntary "hen" parties are the rule of the day. But hen parties, as the sole fare, have never been popular among women, and mixed company in older people provides the semblance of normality with advantages for both and embarrassment for none.

The fate of lesbians in older age is not different from that of any other elderly person. In younger years, the sexual interest of women in women has much of the character of mother and child, as Dr. Helene Deutsch lucidly explained in *Psychology of Women.* Since neither of the two parties can completely fulfill the expectations of the other for any length of time, the intimate side of the relationship here too is rarely permanent. They are not necessarily men-haters; they simply don't want to go to bed with them. If the partners have set up housekeeping together or gone into a joint business, they eventually seek emotional satisfaction outside the home while they continue living together as friends and companions in all but the sexual aspect. In this, they are no different from their counterparts of the opposite sex or, for that matter, from some married couples who have arrived at similar arrangements. For them, as for homosexuals, social contact, friendship, and loyalty are neither age-bound nor sex-bound and can remain active throughout a lifetime. Nigel Nicolson's *Portrait of a Marriage*—the marriage of his parents—beautifully illustrates this statement.

In summing up, we have observed that old people do have emotions just as they did when they were young, and they can find gratifications—perhaps on a more modest and less stormy scale, but gratifications just the same. I would like to add that every person has a right to find happiness in his own fashion.

Nine

MAKING LIFE EASIER AND KEEPING FIT

*T*o make concessions to the
changing conditions of our body as we get older is the simplest
and surest way to cushion the blow and get accustomed to what life
imposes on us from here on out. When in repose and relaxed, an
aged person does not feel any different from the way he has always
felt, yet it would be folly to deny that he has changed. Consequently, his mode of living must change too. Just as bending with
the storm diminishes its impact, gradual changes in the organization of our lives work in the same way.

ADAPTATIONS IN WORK

As time goes on, an aged person may feel that he wants to ease
the burdens and responsibilities he has been carrying, and yet he
still wants to remain active in his chosen field. He might select the
path one physician took. After some years of sharing an office
with another physician in the same specialty, she found that the
economic and professional responsibilities had become too much
for her. Her solution was to give up the partnership and become
her colleague's assistant. In this way, she was able to continue her
life's work, earn a livelihood, and yet be free of a burden that
had become too heavy. Although she must have undergone deep

agony and doubt until she came to the conclusion that this was the best course under the circumstances, she never regretted this decision.

A businessman I know did something similar to prepare for his old age. Having no heir, he sold his business to his employees with the proviso that they would not take over until he had died or reached seventy-five. It was also agreed that in case he was still alive at that age and able to work, he would continue as an adviser to the firm. Neither of these is an isolated occurrence. Quite a number of business people do not want to continue carrying the responsibilities and risks any businessman must accept, but they do want to remain active and play a part in their calling. Compromise makes this possible.

WHEN NOT AT HOME

It is not only careers but also the daily routine that must be altered to reduce the chance of mishaps and accidents on the street and at home. To begin with, activities should be spaced so that no undue fatigue arises. You should make a schedule for each day so that your errands can be grouped in the same vicinity. Local stores should be patronized, in order to eliminate the need for long train, bus, or subway rides. Daily marketing, with smaller loads to carry, may be advisable. This has the advantage of avoiding the need to tire yourself out needlessly by carrying heavy parcels. In addition, it provides an objective for going out every day, which means getting more fresh air and seeing more people than you would if you remained at home.

If possible, do not go out in bad weather, but if you must cope with high wind, sleet, or snow, do not hesitate to ask a younger passer-by for assistance in crossing the street. The safest way to get across a one-way avenue is to use the south side of the side street when the avenue is northbound and to use the north side when the avenue is southbound. Walking with smaller steps and stepping off the curb sideways may prevent an accident. Using a cane often increases stability. You should have no false pride about employing mechanical aids wherever advisable, nor need you feel embarrassment at being seen relying on them. The resulting relief from anxiety as well as pain is ample reward for the admission of weakness, and its value to the old person should never be underestimated.

When you are going out for the evening, you may find that a nap or long rest in the afternoon is helpful. Being refreshed, you will be better company for the people you are with, and you will enjoy yourself more because you will be alert and better able to participate in whatever the program may be.

Do not go out at night unescorted. Apart from the higher risks to personal safety after dark in a city, the street lighting is usually not good enough to guide an old person securely to his destination. Even more important, do not drive a car after dark. You should not drive at all except with the explicit permission of your physician. The reason for this is that some vascular changes occur in the healthiest of old persons. These changes may cause blackouts that last but a fraction of a second but can cause serious accidents endangering not only the life of the driver but also his passengers, other cars, and pedestrians. Besides, the headlights of an oncoming car have a very strong effect on the eyes of the driver, and in later years the adaptation to changes in the intensity of light is slower than it was in earlier years. As a result, you may overlook a second car coming after the headlights of the first have passed or you may not see a person crossing the road directly after.

AT HOME

It has long been established that most accidents occur at home. In older people, they are sometimes caused by tripping because the feet are not lifted high enough while walking or when changing position. Or when getting out of bed or rising from a chair, a slight unsteadiness may occur. The adaptation to the change of position may lag a little because of the general slowing of reaction time in all our movements. You can avoid a mishap by remaining standing for a second or two before starting to move. When getting up from a chair, make sure of your balance before you walk. In short, take your time in whatever you do; do not rush.

Old people should not go about in the dark even in the familiar surroundings of their own bedroom. A person who has awakened from sleep needs time to adjust his sense of direction. This, too, can play us a bad trick when there are no familiar objects to assist us in orientation. For the same reason, do not climb ladders. Moreover, sudden dizziness when craning the neck is not confined to old age. It can happen at any age, but a younger person's coordination is faster, and he can catch his balance more easily and is, therefore, less liable to have an accident.

While carrying a glass or a bottle, you may find it helpful to put your little finger on the bottom so that the object cannot slip from your hand. Mishaps of this kind occur more often in the morning before we have fully regained consciousness after a night's sleep. There should be a hand grip in the bathroom next to the toilet to help in getting up, and another one in the shower to hold onto while standing on one foot and scrubbing the other. There should be a rubber mat or some similar device as a safeguard against slipping. If you do not feel strong enough to get out of the tub from a sitting position, you may feel more secure if you turn around and get up from a kneeling position.

VISION

While reading or using your eyes for any close work, you should have rather intense lighting coming from behind your left shoulder (for a right-handed person). Light coming from the front may blind you momentarily if you inadvertently look directly into it. Regular eye examinations are important; properly prescribed glasses or even surgery can make the difference between living and vegetating.

One of the most frequent eye afflictions in later years is the progressive opaqueness of the lens in one eye or both called cataract. Surgery is the only remedy for this condition. If the eye is otherwise healthy, the operation, dreaded by most people, is a rather simple procedure. It consists of the removal of the deteriorated lens. Modern technology has made the adjustment after the operation so thorough and so helpful that it deserves mention. The lens that has been removed must be replaced by eyeglasses, which, until recently, were of limited help. They enabled the wearer to obtain only tubular vision: he could see only when looking straight ahead; when looking sideways, he therefore had to move his head instead of moving only his eyes. Now we have contact lenses, which are widely used. The individual wearing them can very often achieve normal vision; he can look in any direction simply by moving his eyes as he had done before. The thick glasses that betrayed the fact that a cataract operation had been performed have all but disappeared in public; contact lenses contribute not only to the improvement of vision but also to the improvement of the general demeanor and appearance of the wearer. If you have other impairments of vision, you should see your doctor at regular intervals.

HEARING

It is not an easy job to convince an old person that he—or especially she—is hard of hearing. This information is received almost as an insult. There are various causes for the gradual impairment of hearing, which is much more common than one might assume. Of the population between forty-five and sixty-five, 5 per cent is hard of hearing. This figure increases to almost 13 per cent between sixty-five and seventy-five, and to 25 per cent over seventy-five.

Only a medical examination can determine which kind of treatment offers the greatest promise. Some people are helped by surgery, but where this is not indicated, a hearing aid may be of immeasurable help. Present-day models are so small as to be all but invisible. Yet the resistance against wearing an aid is still as great as when the deaf had to use old-fashioned ear trumpets. And it is this defeatist attitude that is largely responsible for the disappointment that occurs in many instances when a hard-of-hearing person tries to wear a hearing aid. Because of exaggerated expectations of what the instrument can do, he is unwilling to give it a fair test.

A hearing aid is more or less an amplifier. It works like a radio in miniature, catching the sound from the air and bringing it closer to the ear. Like any other radio, it has a limited radius of reception. What it cannot do, but what the unhappy wearer expects it to do, is to discriminate among the sounds it transmits. In our daily lives, we have learned this discrimination from childhood and practice it every minute of the day, without realizing it. The best illustration of this is the young mother who will sleep through the noise of a fire engine roaring past her house, but who will be awake as soon as her baby begins to whimper in the next room. Even under normal circumstances, it is possible to eliminate only a certain portion of extraneous noise. When the noise becomes too loud, we do not hear someone next to us. All this the hard-of-hearing person has to relearn as the deafness progresses. Moreover, the weakening of the ability to hear is accompanied by a dulling of the ability to distinguish various kinds of sounds. An affected person is apt to tell you: "I hear you speak but I do not understand what you are saying." The hearing aid can correct a great deal of this defect, but not all. Only if a person wears the aid all day over a considerable length of time can he regain some of his former ability to tune out part of the extraneous noise.

A well-lighted room will aid not only one's vision but also one's hearing, especially if one faces the speaker. The speaker's facial expression and his gestures are of great help in the interpretation of his words. Where the deafness is such that a hearing aid would not be of any assistance, lip reading can maintain contact with the outside world. To read lips most successfully, a face-to-face conversation is the best, with the one with whom the hard-of-hearing person is talking placed directly in front of him. With practice and a certain adaptability, communication is possible even in groups. If worse comes to worst, the deaf person may keep a notebook and pencil ready to be used by the person with whom he is conversing. Speaking of notebooks, pads handily placed will guard against memory lapses—which are not uncommon in older people.

The hard-of-hearing person would also do well to keep the front door locked and secured by a chain whenever he is alone. And I would advise having a buzzer installed in every room in order not to miss a caller. Do not open the door unless you are sure whom you are admitting. For a nominal charge, your telephone can be equipped with an extra-loud bell and an adjustable amplifier.

KEEPING TO A "TIMETABLE"

In addition to the necessary slowing down of the tempo of living, an older person should also maintain a definite routine of living for the sake of physical comfort. The human body reacts to periodicity and gets out of kilter if its routine is disturbed. Anyone who has traveled abroad and has encountered a time difference will confirm the fact that it takes quite a while to resume one's former rhythm after returning. When we change our mode of living, we should retain a routine, as for instance in getting up in the morning and retiring at night. Diets should be checked with your physician; food fads should be avoided. Proper food and regular eating habits are a much better guarantee of proper elimination than any medication or mechanical devices.

KEEPING UP APPEARANCES

In running your household and taking care of your personal needs, do not try to do the impossible just to prove your independence. You deceive no one but yourself. The personal care of the body— shaving, combing the hair, trimming the nails, and the like—may become difficult or even dangerous when unsteady hands wield a sharp instrument or bad eyesight no longer permits keen focusing. Under those circumstances, it would be advisable to have these chores done for you by somebody else. Under no circumstances should good grooming be neglected. Every old person should appear at his best at all times as much as it is possible to do so. This goes for personal fastidiousness as well as clothing. It is cleanliness that counts, not style. Quite a few old people who have seen better days will prefer to keep on wearing their out-of-style wardrobe rather than to spend money on a new one. Other old people wear hand-me-downs that are also not of the newest fashion. There is no reason why an old person whose income is limited should not make use of this way of cutting down the cost of living, as long as the clothes are in good condition. And many women—and men— know how to use a needle and thread to patch up torn places. Our self-esteem depends as much on our own appearance in the mirror as on the facial expression of an acquaintance we may run into. Letting one's appearance go is the beginning of letting go everywhere else.

COMMON ABUSES OF NUTRITION

To begin with, do not overeat. Old people burn up less energy than young ones because of the slowing-down process inherent in aging. If an old person eats the same quantity of food as he used to when he was working hard, he will put on weight; this in turn will increase the strain on his heart and may also raise his blood pressure. The wrong kind of diet may have other equally damaging consequences, such as vitamin deficiencies and diabetes caused by overloading the body with carbohydrates.

In order to get the most benefit from eating proper food, a person must be able to chew it thoroughly, since the saliva is an integral part of the digestive process. To keep your teeth, be they grown or bought, in good working condition is almost as essential as food itself.

There is a common saying that a swig of liquor before retiring is good for old people. I do not know how this idea sprang up, but it is as good an excuse to have a drink as any other. It may not do harm to anyone with a healthy stomach, but it may cause heartburn in others. You had better check with your doctor before acquiring this habit.

I am almost embarrassed to talk about well-nourished oldsters, because I know that the overwhelming majority of the aged are poor, and, for most of them, proper nourishment is beyond their means. Federal food-stamp programs and the meals available in day centers and similar low-cost opportunities should be taken advantage of by every oldster who cannot otherwise have an adequate diet.

FALSE PRIDE

Some old people become extremely run-down because they do not seek assistance when they first begin to need it. Many of them refuse to apply for public assistance or postpone this step so long that it is almost too late to nurse them back to health; they simply will not admit that they have become unable to look after themselves. Some of them worry that they might embarrass their children if it became known that they were not successful enough to take care of their parents; or they are ashamed to own up to the fact that their children do not care enough to help them. Some others are simply proud.

Recently I saw in consultation an eighty-four-year-old patient in the internal medicine department of the hospital I am affiliated with. I was told that she was suicidal. She had been hospitalized because of a heart condition. Since this is a chronic ailment, her Medicare benefits were running short, but she refused steadfastly to apply for Medicaid, because it meant public assistance. She declared that she would rather kill herself than become a public charge.

This old woman had worked all her life and for many years helped to support her invalid husband. The couple had no children and no living relatives. Before being admitted to the hospital, she had lived in a public-housing project nearby. It was quite impressive to observe how many neighbors visited her regularly in the hospital: young and old, men and women, whites and nonwhites came and were concerned. One of the most faithful was an old man, a contemporary of hers, who visited every day. I frequently saw him feeding her when she was too weak to eat by herself. He explained his interest this way: "When my wife was sick, Mrs. Y. looked after her until she died; now it is my turn to take care of Mrs. Y." Other neighbors told similar stories.

It took some effort on my part to convince her that as a former taxpayer, and especially as a human being, she was entitled to be assisted when she was in need and that her many friends proved that she had earned whatever help she now required. I am glad to report that she finally consented to apply for Medicaid and that she entered an old people's home a few days later. This is just one example of the many old people who postpone asking for aid; quite a few would rather commit suicide and not all of them can be stopped in time.

MEDICAL CARE

The next very important suggestion is: see your doctor at regular intervals. Under normal circumstances, a complete checkup once or twice a year should be sufficient. Wherever possible, have your examination with the same doctor or with the same clinic each time. Sometimes only the comparison of current and previous laboratory tests will tell whether important changes have taken place in the body. It is not a good procedure to change from doctor to doctor. A physician whom you have consulted over a number of years knows you and your condition much better than a new one who does not know what your usual state of health has been.

Do not doctor yourself. Medication that has helped you in the past may not be the right one for you in later years. You may need a different dosage or an entirely different treatment now.

Moreover, medicines that have been kept for a long time deteriorate; they not only may lose their efficacy but may become harmful. Popular medications, such as aspirin, antacids, and the like, are very helpful when taken in small doses, but they can damage the body severely when taken in large amounts over a long period of time. This warning applies to people of all ages.

During the last few years, medicine has been alerted to another reason to exercise care in dosing oneself. Quite unexpected discoveries have been made regarding the effect of drugs on the body: various drugs that were prescribed at the same time for unrelated illnesses have been found to be interacting with each other, thus either augmenting the effect of one or counteracting the effect of another. This means that sometimes dosages have turned out to be wrong, and that the patient's system may have become upset when one or another drug was discontinued after it was no longer needed. Your doctor will know how to mix medications that do not interfere with one another.

For some older people, the remedies of a friend or a sympathetic neighbor or something that has been advertised as a panacea in various media seems to have more allure than a regular prescription given by a physician. Consulting a doctor is like admitting that something is wrong; taking the medication of a friend is less committing. Older persons may refuse to seek professional advice on principle. On more than one occasion, when I suggested that an oldster have a medical checkup, he refused with words like this: "What's the use? When I tell my doctor about my aches and pains, all he has to say is, 'What do you expect? You're not getting any younger.'" Other doctors will be even more blunt and state that old age is an illness in itself. This is a remnant of the lack of medical knowledge of two generations ago. But it is still parroted, especially by physicians who themselves have not come to grips with aging. This unconscious conflict leads to the same prejudice against old people that, to this day, stands in the way of improving their lot in general.

ADJUSTING TO PHYSICAL CONDITIONS

The problem of health does not enter the general picture of aging in the early stages of getting older, but when the individual reaches his seventies, it becomes more difficult to keep protracted illnesses in check.

In most cases, what plagues an old person is not actually old age but systemic diseases, such as arthritis, emphysema, asthma, or intestinal upsets. Special diets and adaptations in the mode of living—giving up smoking, alcohol, sweets, and the like—can help a great deal. Some other disturbances demand such major changes as moving to a warmer climate, which may mean becoming separated from family and friends, as the price for breathing more easily.

These and other measures are personal choices the aging person has to make, and no one has a right to interfere. He should discuss his problem with his spouse and with his friends and his doctor. He can then weigh the pros and cons offered, but the ultimate decision must be his. Some chronic diseases do not represent a threat to life, but are apt eventually to impair the mobility of the oldster. And they may be accompanied by often almost unbearable pain, which diminishes the zest for living and encroaches upon the individual's cherished independence when outside assistance becomes a necessity.

A great many hospitals are engaged in intensive research that is daily discovering new ways to ameliorate the patient's suffering, even if it is sometimes not possible to restore his health. Rehabilitation centers prescribe medications aganst pain while keeping the patient mobile; they also teach the individual how to utilize the mobility he still has and how he may possibly improve it. They also construct special appliances that facilitate the patient's movements, lessen his suffering, and increase his self-reliance.

If an oldster needs assistance in his physical care but is otherwise still self-sufficient, a visiting nurse can be of immeasurable help. This is evident, for instance, in the case of a woman of eighty-five who suffered a stroke that deprived her of the use of one arm. After she was discharged from the hospital, she moved to a hotel for senior citizens at the seashore. There she has engaged a visiting nurse who comes in the morning to help her get up and get ready for the day. The nurse returns in the evening to prepare her for bed. The old woman spends the rest of the day with friends who live in the same hotel, taking short walks and having her meals in their company. As long as it is physically possible, you should keep on taking part in the life around you. Visiting with friends and relatives is an essential activity. If personal visits are not feasible, telephone calls or frequent letters are good substitutes. If your friends are contemporaries, keep in mind that they are probably just as lonesome as you are.

Older people should make every effort to keep up their social contacts, including, if possible, younger people. To be taken on equal terms with the younger generation fills the old one with pride. If he wants this popularity to continue, he should not try to entertain his younger friends with exploits of his own youth. He should leave the bragging to them and remember how bored he was when he was a young man and had to listen to the conquests and adventures of his elders. By the same token, old ladies should not brag about how beautiful they were in their youth, nor should they boast about the men they could have married, who now, in their later years, are rich or famous. To be a good listener is the best way for an old person to be liked by the young.

A hobby is a very useful means for establishing or maintaining relations with family, friends, and others. One cannot always be on the go, and one cannot always sleep.

Reading the papers and listening to the news is as important as food and sleep. Nothing is more demoralizing than losing ties with the world outside. If you cannot be an active participant, as you once were, you can at least remain a spectator. The more a person withdraws into himself, the fewer visitors he will have as time goes on, because there will be less and less to talk about with anyone who drops in. In the end, the visitors will lose interest and stay away.

We should recognize that arranging our lives in accordance with our faculties is just as much a part of successful aging as the need for self-acceptance. By becoming aware of the hazards of living that confront us every day, we learn the ways that are helpful in maintaining our morale and self-confidence.

Ten

THE AGED PARENT AND HIS FAMILY

*T*he strongest ties between people and the deepest feelings of belonging have always lain within the family. Because of the profound changes in our social structure and the trend toward the establishment of separate homes in the four corners of the earth, the concept of the family has shrunk from the tribe and the clan of early days, until it is now restricted almost entirely to parents and their children—as long as the children are too small to fend for themselves. Grandparents are counted as members of the family only when they share the common household. This development clearly demonstrates that something has gone amiss in the relationship between the middle-aged and their elderly parents. The tension between these two generations seems almost as great as the generation gap separating younger parents and their teen-age children.

ROOTS OF THE PARENT-CHILD RELATIONSHIP

The relationship between parents and their adult children is a very complicated one indeed. Whatever happened between them from the birth of the child onward has left its impression on both—on the parent as well as on the child. Most of this has been buried in the unconscious, and if they were confronted with the facts, they would both deny them. There is no human relationship that is not a mixture of love and hate, a truth any mature individual can admit without feeling particularly guilty. Since no one can completely live up to another person's expectations about him in any satisfactory relationship, disappointments and occasional frustrations must accompany even the deepest love. While the immature adult swings from a great deal of hate to a great deal of love and back again whenever he discovers qualities in his beloved that he does not like, the emotionally mature individual learns to live with the personal characteristics of his loved one and arrives eventually at a unified view of the person dear to him. This means that his love and his acceptance of the beloved remain untouched even in the face of some negative qualities, so long as they do not outweigh the positive ones. In other words, it is the individual as he is who is loved and not an idol with feet of clay. A discerning parent in time comes to recognize and respect the fact that his child has an individuality of his own, and has to be taken as an entity and not as a summary of parts.

No such objectivity is at first possible between parents and their small children. It is necessary for the parent to overestimate his child so that he will be willing to make all the sacrifices the baby requires and will accept lifelong responsibility for the child. It is necessary for the child to idealize the parent because he depends for survival not only on the care but also on the good will (love) of the parent. In order for the child not to lose his pride and self-esteem while accepting the many restrictions a parent must impose on him in the process of his integration into the social setting, he must put the parent on a pedestal.

In light of these facts, one can easily understand that throughout their lives both sides will harbor a wealth of feelings of all kinds that are never allowed to come to the surface lest they overwhelm the individual with guilt. The human mind cannot stand a vacuum; if there is a situation that a person cannot explain to himself, he will invent some reason for the occurrence and then take it for the truth. This is the stuff of which prejudice is made. Moreover, magic is an accepted fact in the mind of every child, and it persists to some degree in almost all of us throughout our lives. Without some such form of subterfuge, life would be unbearable, and magic thinking, or fantasy, is the refuge from imprisonment by the necessities of life and from hated routine.

Wishful thinking is at work when parents bring up their children in the way they wanted to have been brought up when they were young. This means that most parents try to rear their children as improved copies of themselves and often overlook the fact that children are people with inclinations and reactions of their own that may be quite different from those of their parents.

In their behavior toward their children, some parents express conflicts between themselves, making the children into the scapegoat, or clinging to them for protection, or confiding in them as if they were adults, and expecting them to take sides. Other parents bring up their children with the motto "Mother [Father] knows best"—stifling initiative and depriving them of developing any appreciable self-reliance. All these manifestations—human as they are—leave their mark on the growing children forever and will influence their attitude toward their parents in later life, as well as toward their own children.

This is a very good opportunity to dispel a myth that has plagued parents and children throughout the ages. It is the assertion that any parent loves all his children equally and that all children feel equal love toward their parents. At least, that is what they are told they must feel, and what parents persuade themselves to feel toward their offspring, while deep down all of them know that this is not the case. By the same token, this is what every parent tells his child when the youngster wants to be assured that he is the favorite. The truth is that some personalities click and some rub each other the wrong way, and it is the same among members of a family. This will also influence the relationship between the generations in old age.

In their later years, some parents take out on their children the conflicts they were unable to resolve in relation to their own parents; and some adult children take unconscious revenge on their aged parents for the "injustices," real and imagined, they suffered from them in earlier years.* Quite a few parents hold it against their children that they rejected the opportunities offered to them, sometimes at great sacrifice. The reason is that children regard opportunities forced upon them as an expression of parental authority and often rebel against them as a matter of principle—even if they would have liked to accept them. It is an old truth that opportunities that are offered on a silver platter are no opportunities at all; they must be earned in order to have effect. A German saying describes this manifestation: "What you have inherited from your ancestors you must earn if you are to own." Although intelligent parents are aware of this, they are nevertheless nostalgic about the opportunities they did not have. Yet one never knows what they would have done with them if they had had them.

IN-LAWS

I have discussed this mechanism in detail, because as the children grow up, some of these conflicts persist or reappear in the form of adolescent difficulties—in the choice of work and of the mode of living. Later they may manifest themselves in the choice of a spouse. Meanwhile, the parents' overexpectation in regard to their children will persist. This is the reason, for instance, why no

* M. R. Kaufman, "Old Age and Aging," *American Journal of Orthopsychiatry*, vol. 10, no. 1 (January 1940).

prospective son- or daughter-in-law is good enough in the eyes of many a parent to marry any child of theirs. It is also a fact that many a younger person repeats his unconscious conflict with his own parents by not getting along with his in-laws. This is also the reason for conflict between the son-in-law and an ambitious mother of the bride, and, conversely, it is why very few old women would want to live in their son's home. Even when the child's marriage turns out well, the guilt feeling in the aged parent over the initial rejection or doubt, as well as the reservation of the bride (or groom) in regard to the future in-laws, is bound to erect a wall between the two parties forever. Evidence of this distance is that quite a few daughters-in-law call their mothers-in-law "Mrs."

THE COUPLE'S PARENTS

If the family members have close contact with each other, the relationship of the grandparents with the grandchildren acquires special significance. In large families, such as are common in some minority groups, the grandchildren are simply taken in by the grandparents one by one and are brought up as if they were younger siblings of their mother or father. In this way the grandmother assumes the role of the mother; as a result, the mother loses some of her authority as a parent, a fact that also contributes to the loosening of the child-parent relationship in later years.

This three-generation family arrangement is frequently entered into for economic reasons. The grandparents' Social Security payment is a welcome addition to a meager family income, and at the same time gives the grandparents a feeling of purpose in life and a sense of dignity, while it leaves the younger adult in the family free to go out to work.

Even if the grandparents retain their own home, their role in the life of a grandchild is unique. The grandparent, fearing isolation and loneliness, wishes to be loved and to be needed and is, therefore, more permissive and liberal with privileges and presents than the child's own parents can afford to be. Grandparents do not have or very rarely assume responsibility for the proper development of the grandchild, while the parent has to shoulder this obligation.

In certain circumstances, the grandparent's role may even be deliberately destructive of family relationships. This is frequently the case with an older woman who has lived without a husband for some time. She learns to regard her oldest or her only son as a substitute for the absent husband, and she uses the grandchildren as pawns in the conflict between herself and her son's wife, whom she cannot forgive for having "taken my son away from me."

A classic example of such a situation is described in *Eleanor and Franklin,* by Joseph Lash. Hoping to avoid relinquishing her son, Franklin, to his future wife, Mrs. Sara Roosevelt tried to postpone the wedding as long as she could. Even after it took place, she did not allow the young couple to lead their own lives. She always regarded her daughter-in-law as an intruder and continued to compete with her for the love of her children. Repeatedly she bribed them with presents and attempted to influence them against Eleanor by telling them that she herself loved them more than their own mother did.

Not all mothers-in-law are so hostile, but a certain fear of the mother-in-law rarely leaves the young wife completely. Visiting mothers-in-law are dreaded by the younger woman, who may feel herself to be perpetually under scrutiny, with her house minutely inspected—including the kitchen, the menu, and, at times, even the number of pieces of soap used.

The son-in-law, in his turn, does not welcome his mother-in-law's visits. A stay planned for a day or two may sometimes last weeks and months and end up with the wife having acquired new ideas about refurnishing the house.

A more humorous explanation is often given for the son-in-law's not infrequent dislike of his mother-in-law: he does not want to know what his wife might look like twenty-five years hence. This and other jokes about mothers-in-law speak proverbial truths; they are funny only when they apply to someone else. But one can easily understand that remnants of these conflicts may flare up and become intensified when the two parties live in close quarters under the same roof, even many years after the wedding.

Rivalry between fathers and sons occurs, too, especially if the two work together. The son is likely to think that his father is no longer an asset to the joint enterprise, while the father may consider himself indispensable.

MULTIGENERATION FAMILIES

The prospect of living together in close quarters sometimes reveals a tragic lack of understanding and empathy between the two or three generations, even if there is a great deal of good will and affection. I remember a woman in her late sixties who did not have sufficient means to maintain an independent household after she became a widow. She had three married daughters with families. Each of the daughters was very sympathetic, and together they offered the following proposal: Mother should spend four months of each year with each daughter. Since the economic situation of these three families was secure but rather moderate, there was no room in any of their homes that could be turned over to the mother. She would have to sleep on the living-room couch. Everyone can see that this was a completely unacceptable solution: no place to relax, no privacy, and no chance to retire in case company stayed late. To boot, there were teen-age children in each family who wanted to entertain their friends in their home. The old woman responded to this "solution" with a depression that disappeared only after arrangements were made for her to move to modest lodgings of her own. Even if the woman could have been given a room of her own, she would still have remained in the role of a boarder who had to change quarters every four months.

It would be futile to try to lay the blame for the tension between the generations at anyone's door. By and large, aged parents and their near-aged children will continue the relationship they had with each other in the early years. But in time, some of the inhibitions have been weakened and true feelings are more readily allowed to come to the surface.

If the two adult generations must share living quarters, there must be a great deal of tact, compromise, and forbearance. It is essential to work out certain modes of living so that both parties retain their identity and social independence. When there is company for the evening, for instance, the parent can and should retire to his or her own quarters soon after the meal is over or even eat in his room. If the oldster wishes to entertain his own friends, this might be done during the daytime, when most of the other members of the household are usually out.

Considerable self-restraint is needed when there are children in the common household. Unless specifically authorized by the parents, a grandparent should not interfere with the way a grandchild is brought up, especially not in the presence of the child. Rearing the child is the parents' job, and the standards of the old person are just as unacceptable to the young as theirs are to the old. It is particularly upsetting to the young to hear the phrase: "When I was your age, I . . ." Times were different then, and moral codes were different, too. Moreover, the old person's memory is sometimes incorrect and sometimes expresses more wishful thinking than fact. Also, one can disapprove without giving oneself as an example.

RESENTMENTS BETWEEN THE GENERATIONS

Many old people are reluctant to air their complaints about their children. They are embarrassed even to admit that things are not so agreeable as they would wish; they try to find excuses for their children's visiting or writing so seldom; they tend to take some of the blame upon themselves. Often they believe that it is only they who have difficulties with their children and that other families live in perpetual bliss. Other oldsters with whom they may compare notes dissemble in the same fashion.

A careful observer can get at the truth simply by watching. For instance, most day centers for the aged arrange for the celebration of national holidays for their members. So that the center can make adequate plans, the members are requested to make their reservations early. It is pathetic to see those who postpone making their reservation until the last possible moment, hoping against hope that an invitation will come from their family.

In addition, some old people are very self-conscious when dealing with their family. They have the feeling that they must not speak their mind lest they offend and even that they must give presents constantly. There is a phrase in German coined by an old person a long time ago: "Schweigen, schlucken, schenken." Freely translated, it means: "Keep your mouth shut and your purse open." In a group-therapy session at a day center for the aged, an old man blurted out: "As long as I was able to give, I was placed at the head of the table. Now I am not even invited."

Some of these feelings of resentment do not seem to be unjustified. Many a parent feels responsible for his child throughout his whole life, and many a child expects this protection irrespective of his age, no matter how clearly logic tells him that since he reached maturity he is no longer entitled to it either legally or morally.

One need only watch adult children visiting their parents'

home. They do not hesitate to ask for a piece of furniture or knick-knack if it strikes their fancy or if they need some particular object. They do not seem to notice that the wall looks bare after they have asked for and taken the picture that had hung there before. I know of a family with two aged parents living in their own home. Their children, near-aged, have come to an understanding among themselves of how they will distribute their parents' belongings after their death. It has not occurred to any of them that the parents might wish to dispose of their things themselves.

In the same vein, a son in his early forties accused his mother of depriving him of part of his inheritance by living in a rented apartment instead of buying a cooperative which would have given him some property after her death, while only the landlord was profiting from his mother's rent.

FINANCIAL ASSISTANCE

Most grown sons or daughters do the best they can; it's just that they are not able to project themselves into the future and cannot understand that an older person has needs, has a right to live, a right to get help from the younger ones. The children sometimes feel that the parent is taking something away from what belongs to them by living as long as he does. Social Security has ameliorated this situation, but only to a very small extent.

Some parents do make demands on their children in later life, but I believe that there are only a few who actually take advantage of their children. On the contrary, the fact that so many parents feel responsible for their children throughout their lives partly explains why old people have submitted up to now so meekly to the treatment they receive from their children and from the younger generation as a whole. They all but apologize for living so long and giving ground for so much trouble.

However appreciative they may pretend to be, some parents

are, at least at times, disappointed in the care and attention they receive. As I said before, no matter how strongly an old person professes to desire independence, he wants and needs the proximity and protection of the younger generation. Parents feel that they have earned it by the care they gave their children when they were small, that they have earned some sacrifices on the children's part through their own self-denials, which were necessary to give the children their chance in life. Yet these children very often feel that the parents' expectations are unreasonable. There is the old saying that one parent can bring up six children while six children cannot take care of one parent. Even if not all complaints on the part of parents are realistic, we will find more often than not that the old ones' charges are not unjustified.

In a study of 890 aged Californians held in the 1950s, 90 per cent stated that their children would be willing to assist them, but only half thought that they would be able to do so. Of the children able to help, approximately one-third urged their parents to apply for public assistance, and two-thirds, "in spite of their ability to help, are ready for others to assume the responsibility for part or all of the support of their parents."*

Yet the children have their side, too. An explanation for these conflicting interpretations of facts can be found in Freud's writings. In an early paper entitled "Three Essays on the Theory of Sexuality," he speaks of the active repetition of a passive experience. Through this mechanism the child gains mastery over a trauma—for instance, the first trip to the dentist's office, after which the child will repair the teeth of the younger siblings and of everyone else he can lay his hands on; or when playing school, every child wants to be the teacher who "dishes it out," and none wants to play the child who has to take it.

* Floyd A. Bond and The Social Science Research Center of Pomona College, *Our Needy Aged* (New York: Holt, 1954).

Applying this to the parent-child relationship, we see that the adult child repeats actively in his behavior toward his own small children whatever he received from his parents when he was a child. Without this mechanism, it would be incomprehensible that young people—men and women—are willing to have children, to undertake the responsibility for their care and for their future. No mother would be willing to get up during the night to tend to the baby unless something in her unconscious reminded her of the care she received from her mother. The present-day generation of young people is less inclined to raise a family because they have not had this experience with their own mothers. Having "paid this debt" to their own children, young parents today do not feel that they owe anything to their aged parents, while the oldsters expect some return for their early sacrifices.

One other observation seems to bear out this postulate: unmarried and childless children usually maintain a closer relationship with their aged parents and more readily shoulder responsibility for them in their old age than do children who have families of their own. As a matter of fact, the time is not long past when an unmarried child, especially a daughter, was expected to stay with the parents and take care of them as long as they lived.

I would like to emphasize that I have met quite a number of middle-aged people and their aged parents who have a very warm and relaxed relationship to each other. I am sure they arrived at this harmony in adult life after many painful compromises. Good human relationships rest on mutuality and not on obligation.

Yet it cannot be denied that children and their parents today are often not very well acquainted with each other. The pressure of living and the tempo of of our times make everybody hurry from pillar to post; the children have a tight schedule of school, sports, and other extracurricular activities. The parents, too, are busy with their own affairs. Fathers are at the office engaged in the "rat race," and mothers are trying to keep house, supervise the children, and pursue their own interests. Television is allowed to take the place of face-to-face communication, and common relaxation and activities as a family have all but disappeared from the scene. As a result, the children know their parents mostly as providers and sometimes as disciplinarians. No wonder that when they meet later in life, they talk past each other instead of to each other. This calls to mind an exchange between a middle-aged woman and her newlywed young daughter. The older one said: "I want to be your sister." The younger one replied: "I do not need a sister. I need a mother."

PARENTS' AGING

There is one element in the relationship between the aged parent and the near-aged children that has not been sufficiently appreciated in its psychological implications and social consequences. That is the emotional difficulties the near-aged child has seeing the parent decline in his later years. The small child derives his strength from the strength and support he receives from the parent, and some of this dependence never quite disappears. To see the strength of the parent diminish represents a threat to the child, no matter what his age. In addition, seeing the parent weaken reactivates old conflicts and influences the child's course of action in the care and attention he gives to the parent. Some will intensify their solicitude, infantilizing the parent and thus unintentionally increasing the helplessness of the aged, which, in turn, hastens his decline. Others are so shaken that they cannot face watching the process of decline; these children take refuge in neglect. This can, on occasion, be observed when the patient is hospitalized with a terminal disease or mental deterioration. At first, the visits are frequent, but as the parent gets sicker and weaker, and as the hope for recovery diminishes, the visits become rarer and rarer, and sometimes the parent is left to die alone.

CHERISHING INDEPENDENCE

One of the unexpected phenomena of aging is the fierce desire of most aged persons for independence. When they themselves were young, there was no question in their minds that their aged parents would share their home when the time came. Any other arrangement was regarded as a disgrace to the family reputation and had to be avoided at all cost. Only one exception was acceptable to the aged: to have the child and his family move in with the parents. In this way, the old people were protected but remained the head of the household. In some European countries, a small house was built very close to the main house and connected to it with a covered passageway. The old couple moved into the *Stoeckli,* as this refuge was called in Switzerland. This enabled them to retain their freedom, but there was always someone within calling distance in case help was needed.

Yet as the oldster gets still older and his strength wanes little by little, the need to lean on someone stronger than himself comes more and more to the fore. The old one wants the protection of the younger but at the same time wants his independence. In short, he wants to live *near* his child but not *with him.* This need persists even if the aged and their near-aged children get along very well with each other, as most of the two generations do.

As long as both parents are still alive and living together, the question of sharing a home with a child and his family hardly ever comes up. Even if health is failing, each spouse derives a great deal of satisfaction in caring for the other and takes pride in still being useful and being needed. As a matter of fact, investigation has shown that "there was a definite tendency for the older persons who lived in their own homes to be better adjusted than persons who lived in the homes of their children."* Whether the children like it as well is an open question. As for instance, I recently talked with a ninety-year-old woman who had just begun to be in need of assistance because of beginning senility and physical weakness. She lived in moderate but secure circumstances in the apartment she had shared with her husband until he died a few years before, at a ripe old age. After his death, her only daughter moved in with her. The latter, a divorcee, held a responsible full-time job, although with moderate pay. When I casually asked the old lady whether she lived with her daughter, she caught me up sharply, saying: "No, my daughter lives with me." At no time did she let the daughter forget that it was her home that the daughter shared and that she was, therefore, expected to look after her mother.

Wherever and whenever the single aged parent can maintain his or her independence, the relationship with the near-aged offspring will be a far more harmonious one. The near-aged feel a deep respect for the parent who continues to function normally and to maintain his individuality. There is neither condescension nor resentment in their relationship. The good relationship will continue even if the old one becomes financially dependent on his or her children. A few examples may illustrate this point:

One woman (who lived to be a hundred and one!) owned her own home. However, she was supported by a daughter, who lived some distance away and visited her mother, to whom she was deeply devoted, only twice a year. These visits were always made the occasion for celebrations, parties, and festivities. At the end of about two weeks, both had tired of each other and there was an

---

* Gordon F. Streib and Wayne E. Thompson, "The Older Person in a Family Context," in *Handbook of Social Gerontology: Societal Aspects of Aging*, ed. Clark Tibbitts (Chicago: The University of Chicago Press, 1970), p. 463.

affectionate good-by. The daughter admired her mother for keeping her independence and never soliciting any additional visits or financial help.

Another old woman had to be placed in a private nursing home by her only daughter because the younger woman was the wage earner for both of them and could not take care of her aged mother at home. The old woman was very gracious in her insight and understanding of her daughter's predicament. The nursing home was a small one catering to a few "paying guests." The old lady quickly made herself at home, helping with the household chores as best she could. She took on some work (industrial knitting) and earned her spending money in this fashion, so that her daughter had no expenses other than the cost of the boarding. In this way, the mother retained her independence and her self-respect and won the love and respect of everybody who knew her.

In another case, a woman who had been a librarian kept up her special interests and continued working as a free-lancer in her field. At the age of eighty-two, she was asked to come back by the library, where she is currently working from nine to five on special projects. Her two married children, both with families and in strained financial situations, do not expect help from her nor are they able to give any. The relationship is free of frustration or disappointment on both sides. There is unbounded admiration on the children's part for their mother's "spunk," and she, in turn, feels completely independent of them.

Things are not always so clear-cut, and the aging person in her need to be assisted and protected is sometimes the victim of greed or callousness, even on the part of her own children, as these stories show:

W. E. was left a widow when in her eighties. She had always been dominated by her husband. He left her an adequate annuity and the royalties from his writings. Her two sons persuaded her that she did not need more than her annuity and that the royalties should be made over to them. Soon her elder son moved into her apartment with his wife, and the other son reluctantly invited her from time to time for a few weeks. When she required professional care, she was sent to a decidedly second-rate home, where she was treated as a pauper until her death at ninety-six.

F. T. had lived with a widowed daughter, who supported her. Unexpectedly the latter died, and another married daughter, who was well off, took her into her home. The mother lost her household and her sense of security. She felt that she was treated like an intruder and became depressed, and her mental decline was hastened.

THE PARENT'S REMARRIAGE

The adult children's reaction to the remarriage of a near-aged or aged parent varies according to the circumstances and depends most often on the kind of mate the parent selects. If the prospective partner belongs to an age group that is commensurate to the age of the parent and to a comparable social station, there is usually no objection, and even satisfaction. The parent now has a mate, somebody to look after him, to provide company, and the moral and sometimes also the economic responsibility is either removed or diminished. This will be the case particularly if the children and the parent live at great distances from each other.

If, however, there is a discrepancy in age and a suspicion that the oldster has been accepted by the younger one for ulterior motives, then the objection of the family does not seem to be unjustified. A marriage of such uneven partners does not hold much promise for lasting success. The resistance of the family can sometimes be overcome—especially if the parent is financially well off—by a compromise such as this: the marriage is entered into only after a marriage agreement has been signed stipulating that the new mate's inheritance is dependent on the number of years the couple remains married. While in the first case the personal relationship can become warm and friendly, in the second case, the new mate rarely becomes a member of the family.

Parents often have a hard time with their children, and children chafe equally under parental authority. Man's personality is rather complicated in structure, and the sources for conflict intensify the closer the contact between individuals is. Yet when the chips are down, they close ranks and help each other to the best of their ability. The few exceptions need not discourage us from reaffirming the fact that the closest ties a person can have are rooted in the family.

Eleven

LIVING ARRANGEMENTS

TAKING A FLING AT FREEDOM

$\mathcal{W}$hen those of us who are aged today were born, the new grandmother was a very busy person. During the lying-in period, whether at home or in a maternity hospital, Grandmother was called in to run the household and take care of the older children. Afterward she was asked to stay until the young mother could resume her usual duties. These demands kept a middle-aged woman with several children rather busy, and she and her husband were also expected to baby-sit when one of the younger generation took an evening off or went on vacation without the children. By the time these attentions were no longer needed, the grandmother had become an old lady.

With the growing tendency of children to break away from parental authority, surprising changes took place in parents too. I came to realize this some years ago when a woman told me about a conversation she had had with her married daughter. When the young woman spoke about having children, her mother said: "I want you to know that you can't count on me for baby-sitting. Your father and I have different plans." Nowadays, baby-sitting is a part-time occupation for teen-agers and very old people, and the grandparents of today not only accept the new form of family but very often welcome it.

The family, as we oldsters knew it, included the parents,

grandparents, children, uncles, aunts, and cousins of all kinds. And the grandparents' home was the center of family gatherings at Christmas and Thanksgiving, for anniversaries, and the like. In this way, family cohesion was maintained even if the members lived some distance apart. No such center exists today. When the children leave the house and move to different localities, they get married and raise their families without ever meeting their close relatives. Unless the grandparents live in the same household, they are not even considered members of the family.

Government statistics show that almost three-quarters of all couples sixty-five and over live apart from their children. Of the 25 per cent who do share their home with their children, 22.6 per cent remain heads of the household, which means that the children live with them and not they with the children. Should a parent lose a spouse for whatever reason, 69.3 per cent of the fathers and 54.7 per cent of the mothers prefer to live alone. Again, of the parents who share a home with their children, 11.7 per cent of the fathers and 33.0 per cent of the mothers remain heads of the household, retaining not only the authority but also the responsibility and privileges of being the master or mistress of the house.

These figures prove that parents overwhelmingly desire to retain their independence. It may be that even more would do so were it not that, when the widowed or divorced parent becomes unable to live alone, he or she may be forced to move in with one of his children or another relative. Many of the reasons for the unwillingness of both sides to live together as adults were considered in the last chapter. Whatever the reasons are, the trend toward separate living has been growing for the past several decades. It does not start when the parents begin to get old but makes itself felt as soon as the children are ready to leave school or go to work. In other words, the desire to put an end to living under one roof is mutual. Not only do the children want to shift for themselves, the parents also want to be free. They have remained younger and healthier than former generations and are eager to stop being parents. They desire to become people in their own right.

Taking It Easy.   Social Security and pensions have given parents greater economic independence. In the past, they held on to whatever they had been able to save in order to leave their children a nest egg. But since the children can also count on pensions or the like to guarantee them economic security in old age, the parents' incentive to provide for them has lessened, and parents have become more willing to spend their income as they receive it. By the same token, more children do the same with their own resources, regardless of the needs of their parents.

While in 1960, 46.8 per cent of the male labor force sixty-five and older and 11.9 per cent of females in this age group were still holding jobs, by 1971 the figures had dropped to 25.5 per cent of the male and 9.5 per cent of the female workers in the same age group.* This shift indicates that older people are accepting retirement more easily than they used to and are making the most of their new freedom. A great many are now ready to experiment with new modes of living, which explains in part their unprecedented mobility and their interest in the new idea of retirement living.

Ten years ago, there was still a good deal of doubt about experimenting with this possibility. Today the concept of a complete change of environment and of simplified methods of living is taken for granted. The expectation that there are a good many years of living ahead makes planning for a new life more interesting and more important. The kind of living the retirees select depends on two major conditions. One is the financial aspect, which deter-

* *Current Population Reports*, U.S. Department of Commerce, Series P-23, no. 43, February 1973.

mines the standard of living, and the other is the mode of living that the couple or the single person wants. If the oldsters seek company and planned activities, there are several varieties of community living to choose from. If they have special hobbies and interests of their own, company and planned activities will be of less importance than the opportunity to follow their avocations, which will help determine where to establish their new quarters.

Retirement Villages. Retirement residences have developed from simple beginnings in the mid-1930s until now, when they have become a major part of the real-estate industry. One of the first retirement villages was established by the Loyal Order of Moose in Florida. When I first did research into this subject, twenty-five years ago, this organization told me that their retired members lived free of charge in a village where the order owned a number of houses, each accommodating eight to ten people. The household duties, including cooking and maintenance of the premises, were taken care of by the members themselves, in easy stages. I was most impressed by this arrangement, because it kept the old people busy, preserved their self-respect through their contribution to the group, and offered a mode of living closest to that of a family.

Among the buildings in the center of the village was one used for medical purposes and called the Clinic. Initially, the management had been disappointed because so few people came to the Clinic, and then only in an emergency. One day, the name was changed from Clinic to Health Center, and the miracle happened. It became the most popular place in the village. Such is the power of suggestion!

For the Well-to-Do. From these simple beginnings evolved the luxurious arrangements for the well-to-do, along with more modest versions for the average citizen. According to the advertisements for the "leisure villages" that have sprung up in almost every county in the United States, anyone who moves to such a village has the right to expect to spend the rest of his life in perpetual bliss. In order to ensure congeniality among the people in the community, the prospective customer must have money and must not be too young to fit into the group and therefore, as a rule, one person of the couple that joins the community must be no younger than fifty.

The villages consist of two kinds of structures: cooperative individual houses and apartments that may be rented or bought in high-rise buildings. Members are offered manifold attractions— swimming pools, tennis courts, golf courses, country-club living, proximity to shopping centers, movies, restaurants, night clubs, and medical facilities. In addition, there are usually a beauty parlor and a barbershop on the premises, and a chiropodist and a dentist in the vicinity, so that the oldster can have care and comfort without much exertion. These "villages" are located within easy reach of a larger community, with all the conveniences it affords. One can well imagine why the maintenance costs must be rather high, and why membership is beyond the reach of many elderly people.

Middle-Level Facilities.   There are also housing projects for the aged financed in part by the government or by religious or social organizations, which make the cost considerably lower for prospective tenants. These are, however, still few in number, and the waiting lists are usually long.

Since the buildings in these categories are intended for the use of the aged, quite a few adaptations are introduced to make their residents' lives safer and more comfortable, and to reduce the chance of accidents. Wherever possible, there are ramps instead of stairs and nonslip floors. The bathtubs are low so that even a feeble person can lift his foot high enough to get in and out, and grab bars are installed in the tub and next to the toilet to help the oldster sit down and get up. There are special locks for safety. Electrical outlets and shelves are placed at heights that enable the old person to avoid bending down to the floor or climbing a ladder to reach them.

Mobile-Home Parks. A new and more economical way of independent living for the aged population is slowly coming into its own—living in a mobile home. Up to now, trailers were used by youthful travelers, who braved the wind, foul weather, and wet earth that were part of this kind of life. Or they were used by construction workers who lived in a trailer camp in the vicinity of the work site only until their job was finished.

Recently, I learned that living permanently in a mobile-home park is a very satisfactory solution for retired people with limited means. This information came to me from a couple in their early seventies who had purchased a double trailer and parked it in the mobile-home park. Actually, these trailers are not mobile at all; they are cemented into the ground at an angle to each other that provides spacious and comfortable living quarters, as well as privacy. The owner of the park charges a modest amount for the use of the space, garbage removal, and utilities.

My informants had spent their first winter there and liked it very much. Everybody in the camp knew everyone else, yet individual privacy was not infringed upon. Markets were near, as were movies and eating places, and many tenants formed car pools to save money and gas.

One other point should not be overlooked. Attractive as the new communal living in any retirement setting may be, it does represent complete self-exile from past associations. Most of these new domiciles are far away from the inhabitants' former homes, and contact with family and friends is therefore confined to infrequent visits and telephone conversations. Few young people are seen, and then only from a distance, and children are a real rarity. With effort, this drawback can be overcome. As one old person stated: "When you go to town shopping, you meet people of all ages and all kinds, so I do not feel isolated."

Susan R. Sherman, who interviewed this oldster, mentions that the point of satisfaction most often cited in these retirement settings was that the people who move there find and make new friends.* She did not go into the psychology of this surprising statement. One would assume that there are other advantages that make a move pleasant, such as the climate or freedom from household chores. I have pondered this question and asked myself what is really different in the new home that makes it so much more attractive and reassuring, consciously or unconsciously, than the former one. I believe the answer is this: among the many drawbacks of the old place was that the elderly couple became more and more isolated; family members and friends died or moved away, and contact with their children dwindled. Each new death, each old friend who moved away, widened the gap between them and their accustomed world.

In any retirement community, people also move away and die. But no sooner does a vacancy occur than it is filled by someone else moving in. The new acquaintances, close as they may have become, do not leave the same gap as does the death of a friend of a lifetime, and the successor is accepted with the same superficiality as a new shipmate on a cruise with whom the ties do not acquire any depth but remain on a temporary basis. In other words, since they can maintain continuity with the living, the fear of death is put off a little longer.

As long as husband and wife remain healthy, living in one of these communities may be the answer to the enjoyment of retire-

* "Satisfaction with Retirement Housing," *Aging and Human Development*, vol. 3, no. 4 (November 1972), 339–66.

ment, especially if the setup offers various activities. No planning is needed, and boredom can easily be averted. Should one spouse become sick, the other can look after him or her for quite a while until other measures have to be taken. For obvious reasons, seriously incapacitated people are not very welcome in these retirement villages.

Senior Citizens' Hotels.   Other senior communities evolved quite accidentally. Originally, they were fashionable hotels in resorts that catered to the well-to-do elderly who followed the sun in winter or escaped the hot city during the summer. These guests remained at the same hotel for the entire season while younger people came only for shorter vacation periods. As newer and more luxurious hotels were built, these older hotels gradually became permanent homes for the elderly. They are now inhabited almost exclusively by the aged.

Quite a number of onetime resort buildings are being converted to this new purpose. Private manors at the seashore and medium-sized hotels in both cities and suburbs are now used as such residences. They have become very popular among old people with small incomes who live alone; since these places are not adapted for keeping house, they seldom attract couples. But their existence has greatly eased the demand for accommodations in old people's homes.

Among the reasons for the new popularity of the senior citizens' hotels is the fact that they do not carry the stigma of a home for the aged. Also they cost considerably less. (These senior citizens' hotels must not be confused with the senior citizens' residences that are part of most general geriatric institutions.)

The inhabitants of these hotels are entirely on their own; it is up to them to determine the kind of nourishment they take, the kind of life they lead, the kind of care they take of their person, and the kind of medical attention they seek. The buildings and the way in which they are managed are not supervised by any state authority; the reverse is true of all homes that cater to the aged on a business basis. Building codes for these hotels are more lax— a fact that does not always work to the interest of the people who live there.

Some of these hotels are but a step above the so-called welfare hotels. The conditions under which a good many of the aged inhabitants of these places live have been movingly described in recent publications, such as *Nobody Ever Died of Old Age,* by Sharon R. Curtin. Fortunately, the authorities are trying to remedy their worst disadvantages.

Take Your Time. If somebody has stayed in one place for many years and is suddenly forced to move, with the prospect of going to smaller quarters, he may easily become panicky and be apt to make hasty decisions "just to get it over with." This makes him easy prey to high-pressure salesmanship. Advertisements promising paradise and other advantages that cannot possibly be provided induce some old folks to be taken in without thinking the whole project through. The newspapers frequently carry reports of such misrepresentations, yet they do not manage to warn off numerous old people. I cannot stress too strongly that the small print of any contract should be studied very carefully, possibly under expert scrutiny, by people of all ages before signing. And I definitely advise that the new environment be tested by renting for a least one year before a definite commitment is undertaken. It would also be helpful if you can talk to a few people who have been living in the prospective place for some years and who can give you objective information. Moreover, knowing some people in the area you are moving into would make life less lonely, at least at the beginning.

Adjustments have to be made no matter where you go, and no place, however desirable, will fulfill all your expectations—at least until you get used to the new environment, which may take a long time. You will have to meet and adapt to new companions, learn their way of life, acquire hobbies—which may be particularly hard for a person who has been used to a regular working routine and has not had time to develop any kind of diversions or hobbies. One also has to get used to the new standard of living, to the new clothing styles people of leisure are sporting instead of the usual business suit, and to other compromises that go with living in a new group.

SEEKING A HAVEN

Most people in their sixties and early seventies are still active and spry. Yet, time goes on, and once the middle seventies have been passed, age cannot be ignored any longer, especially not if accompanied by protracted illness. The oldster may still not feel old while relaxing in a low chair involved in a stimulating conversation or reading a book that holds his interest. But when he wants to get up, he can almost not make it unless he can hold on to something that steadies him and aids the muscles of his thighs to lift him out of the chair. Unscrewing a bottle top becomes a major project, and bucking the wind while crossing the street is downright hazardous. In other words, it is the physical strength that is diminishing and making it hard for him to continue his accustomed and cherished independence.

What can an aged person do who becomes infirm or sick, but is not sick enough to want to be or have to be placed in a nursing home or to seek admission to an old people's home? And what is he to do if he is not eligible for Medicaid, but cannot continue living without some help? Fortunately, there are quite a few ways for him to make his life more comfortable. The most natural move would be to seek a haven in the home of a child or other relative. This is not an easy step to take, but in many cases, the family is on good enough terms with their oldster to take him in, at least for the time being. If no family member is experienced enough to tend to the old person, it will be necessary to resort to a home-nursing service. There are agencies that send trained nurses on a regular basis to private homes to help with the care of an old person, particularly in the morning and at bedtime. A housekeeper can be hired through state employment agencies all over the country. In other instances, a baby-sitter is of great help, especially to relieve the family members of constant watch and make it possible for them to go to work or have some time for relaxation themselves. The old person can be educated and learn to be alone part of the day and do things for himself, if possible. He can also learn to respect the right of the family members to have some free time and not to take it amiss when they make use of it.

Montefiore Hospital in New York City has initiated a new method of looking after the sick and the aged that is called a "coordinated home-care program." Several other institutes have also applied this system. It offers assistance in a variety of medical, nursing, and social services. In fact, it represents an extension of the hospital into the community, furnishing all necessary services without confining the patient to the hospital. It thus increases the number of beds available for hospital patients. The advantages are that the patient remains in familiar surroundings; he has the care and attention of those closest to him; and when the doctor visits, he is not distracted by other demands—all of which are conducive to a more favorable response to the care he receives, and at much less expense.

The Montefiore system has been imitated all over the world. But regrettably, this and other similar projects are being carried out only on a very limited scale; the tempo of official agencies is notoriously slow, and there is a dire shortage of trained personnel to handle the number of people who need this assistance. There is, however, a ray of hope: a larger number of people are being trained in the nursing of the aged, and many mature and middle-aged women are showing interest in devoting their time to professional geriatric care.

If a family cannot take in an aged member and give him the attention and help he needs, another method can be used: the organization called Foster Home Care, which arranges for a family to take in one or two old people and look after them as if they were members of the family. Social service agencies keep check on the way the old people are treated, in the same way as they do with foster homes for children. The old person's Social Security payments, and assistance from the subsidizing organization, help to finance this project.

Closely akin to this are family-type nursing homes, which provide a real home atmosphere for their paying guests. Located mainly in the suburbs and smaller communities, they charge considerably less than do the large nursing homes. However, this kind of nursing home cannot be expected to work toward its patients' rehabilitation. All it can furnish is good custodial care. Illnesses have to be treated by the local physicians or hospitals.

The real problem that faces the old one and his family is to decide which of the existing facilities would offer the best solution for the care of an aged person. Compromises have to be made here also, because of the diversity of the individual's needs, the large number of applicants, and the relative scarcity of good facilities. The present trend is to place an old person who needs extended or even permanent care in a large institution for the aged. There are two kinds of institutions to choose from: old people's homes and proprietary nursing homes.

Geriatric Centers. Old people's homes, recently renamed geriatric centers, have been greatly modernized and have expanded services to their clientele. Since most of them are maintained by philanthropic and religious organizations, they are able to subsidize a portion of the cost of the resident's care, if needed.

Until a few years ago, their residents consisted of three kinds of old people: the healthy aged, invalids, and those made sick or disabled by age and in need of twenty-four-hour medical and nursing care. Consequently, the services provided were adapted to the specific needs of each category. They are: the residences, the health-related facilities, and the section used as a nursing home.

In the residences, the old people have their own quarters, often in a separate building nearby, with a common living room and common dining room, whose food is furnished by the home. The house physician supervises the residents' health. Residents may come and go as they please; some even have part-time jobs or do volunteer work, and a great many pay their way either fully or at reduced rates, according to their ability. Sometimes their children contribute a portion of the cost, even though in some states they are not legally under any obligation to do so but regard this as their duty or as an expression of their desire to share the responsibility for their aged parents.

The majority of the residents are people who have neither sufficient strength to live alone nor sufficient means to pay for trained private care on the outside. An old person who was accepted as a subsidized resident used to turn over all his assets, including his life insurance, to the home. In turn, for his lifetime, he received full maintenance, including medical and nursing care, a small stipend for spending money, clothing, and miscellaneous items. He was allowed to keep small presents from friends or relatives. In case he changed his mind and wanted to leave, the unspent portion of his assets would be refunded to him.

If a resident needs medical attention, he or she is treated by a member of the home's medical staff, either as an ambulatory patient or in the infirmary. If the illness is more serious, he is transferred to a hospital, very often a teaching hospital with which the home is affiliated.

After his recovery, he is taken back to the home. There he is first placed in a health-related facility, which is the term now used to designate what was formerly called a convalescent home. It serves people who have recovered sufficiently to do without constant medical supervision in a hospital, yet are not well enough to return home or to their usual environment. A patient's stay at a convalescent home is temporary, but critically important. Medical research has found that a long stay in a hospital is less conducive to the recovery of any patient than transfer to a health-related facility as soon as the acute stage of the illness has passed. Consequently, the patient is mobilized as fast as possible and taught to utilize to the fullest whatever physical assets he may still have. After this period, the aged is returned to the residential portion of the geriatric center, whenever feasible.

Numerous programs are developed by occupational therapists to keep old people in contact with life and with other people and to give them an interest in living, even to the extent of having them help in the care of the less fortunate residents.

Once an old person is accepted into an old people's home, he has protection for life. In spite of the fact that the patient sometimes contributes all he owns to the home, it is generally not enough to cover the total cost of taking care of him—even if he spends enough of his assets to become eligible for Medicaid. This is fully explained to the oldster when he applies for admission, and yet some feel that they would rather not avail themselves of the benefits the home can offer; they hesitate to "sign away all I have." They prefer to eke out a miserable existence in independent surroundings, as we have seen earlier, until they are so ill and feeble that they have to be taken to the hospital to die.

From the Residents' Point of View. Life in an old people's home is accepted by the residents in different ways, in keeping with their former standards of living and their various personalities. On the whole, they adjust to it after a while because of the pervasive feeling of protection.

Some criticisms are unavoidable because they are inherent in the situation. The rooms are designed for double occupancy, and some of the new people miss their privacy. One of the residents who had been in such a home for three years explained to me: "You have to be here for ten years before you rate a room by yourself." If the resident's finances permit it, however, single rooms are available from the start. One innovation is that couples are now assigned a room together; in the past, the sexes were separated even if married.

Other reasons for discontent concern two unrelated categories: food and children. The complaints about food are not confined to old people's homes; nursing homes and any other place where oldsters are taken care of also receive these criticisms. There are two reasons that old people do not savor food the way they used to when they were making their own meals: cooking for large groups must be standardized, and it must be rather on the bland side because most old people's stomachs do not tolerate highly seasoned food. In addition, the sense of taste changes with time, as was explained in Chapter 2.

Complaints about children, unfortunately, could fill a chapter of their own. Some of them are extremely attentive but not attentive enough to satisfy the expectation of the lonely parent. Most prospective residents realize the necessity for entering the old people's home but do so only reluctantly. Once there, most of the old folks assure their children that they are content. At first the children visit often and are quite concerned about their parent's well-being. Gradually, however, they begin to go about their usual businesses, and the visits to the parent become fewer and fewer.

I recently talked to a very alert and kind woman of eighty-nine. She had entered the home voluntarily four years before, after the death of her husband. Unlike most of the others in the home, she praised the attention she was receiving from her children, so I encouraged her to give me details. She said: "I have three children. The oldest is a professional man, very busy; he calls me on the telephone every day. But he doesn't have time to come to see me in person. The second one is a salesman; he works six days a week, and when he is free, naturally he has to accompany his wife to do errands. The third is a daughter whose husband is sick, and she has her hands full at home. I cannot expect her to come to see me." In other words, although all of them are fond of their mother and all of them live in the same city, they come to see their mother only on rare occasions. It is pathetic that a woman of this advanced age is reduced to communicating with her children for a few minutes a day by phone.

Some others dissociate themselves from their parents much more drastically. I remember one instance where a son living in the same city as his parent had not visited him for ten years. When the visit finally was made, it was initiated by the social service department of the old people's home where the parent resided.

On the whole, the family's loss of interest becomes even more pronounced when the parent becomes senile and enters dotage. In such instances, the children are so shaken by the change that has befallen the parent that they avoid seeing him and appear only when the end is near.

With the emergence of senior citizens' hotels, the population of old people's homes has undergone a drastic change. As we have

already noted, old people who are still able to look after themselves, however precariously, do not want to enter a home. They
prefer to stay in a senior hotel as long as they can manage it
physically. Consequently, different kinds of oldsters now seek admission to an old people's home: those who are very ill and require
twenty-four-hour medical-nursing supervision; the severely immobile, who are in wheelchairs or who cannot get in or out of bed
without assistance; and the mentally impaired, who for organic
or psychogenic reasons become confused, have severe memory loss,
and are a danger to themselves and others. In other words, old
people's homes have come to resemble nursing homes. The difference is that the latter are proprietary (that is, they are run for
profit) and do not always offer the same quality of care as do the
old people's homes, which are subsidized by public contribution.
While some nursing homes are very well run and give their charges
excellent care, their owners are no different from any other businessmen. There are honest and less honest businessmen in every
branch of industry.

Private Nursing Homes. While the family-type nursing home
provided mainly custodial care, the patients were, on the whole,
not badly treated. But as the homes expanded not only in numbers
but also in size, the resident was treated more and more imper-
sonally until he became simply a number. He had a bed, usually
one or more roommates, nothing to do, no diversions, and few
visitors. He vegetated there until the end came. Often these homes
were located on the outskirts of town, where lack of public transportation, or of any alternative provided by the home, made it difficult for visitors to come and for the resident to keep up his contact with the outside world.

The recent sudden expansion in nursing homes resulted from
the introduction of Medicare and Medicaid. Now that the government underwrote the resident's support, many old people who

would have been unable to afford the cost before could be admitted to these homes.

Because these proprietary nursing homes multiplied so rapidly, they were often neglectful of safety measures and accorded deplorable treatment to the old people. The interest in making money outweighed all other considerations and led to a number of shady practices. To sound a warning against making a "deal" with the management might be in order. Some managers are honest and some are not, and it is safer not to take chances. The following example may illustrate the point: in 1971, a former patient, then eighty-four years old, who had moved to warmer climates, asked me to come south and help her select a nursing home where she could spend the rest of her life. She had become so feeble that she needed permanent nursing care. In canvassing possible places, I visited one that had been highly recommended. I found a very well-kept building; the ground floor was spotless, and the rooms I was shown there were in good condition. I was not shown the upper floors and decided to insist on seeing them too, after I had my talk with the manager. She specified the monthly fee, which was the usual amount charged at that time. To whet my appetite, she mentioned that if the client paid for one year in advance, the charge would be reduced by 10 per cent. This sounded like a sizable concession, especially since I had not expressed any objection to the charge cited, but it occurred to me that the real saving would be only 5 per cent, since money in a savings account would earn 5-per-cent interest anyway.

The manager continued her high-pressure sales talk: if the client paid for two years in advance, there would be no other charges for as long as the old lady lived. My suspicion was aroused, and I remained silent, waiting for more. She went on to tell me that in that case, the fee for medical services would be waived also. I wondered who would be the judge of the need for medical attention—the patient or the management. Before I had a chance to raise this point, which in my opinion was crucial, the cat was let out of the bag: there would be no refund if the client died before the prepayment had been used up. The remainder would be considered a contribution to the general fund of the institution. One cannot avoid the suspicion that there might have been ways and means to see to it that a good portion of the prepayment was left to "the general fund." Just for the record, my patient decided to remain in her own home with the assistance of a practical nurse. She died a natural death five months after my visit.

Under the prodding of Ralph Nader and his associates and other concerned and well-informed people, the ills of the nursing homes became public knowledge. Since the government was the mainstay for the support of the aged poor through Medicaid, it established regulations for the safety and proper care of nursing-home residents. Because the demand for beds far outweighed the supply, the government was at first forced to relax its stringent standards. But it did so in the expectation that improvements would gradually be made in existing homes and that the new ones would be built and run on modern principles. However, the greed of the new industry has been such that these expectations were only rarely fulfilled.

Finally, the government tightened its hold over these homes by more frequent inspections. As a consequence, a number of smaller homes relinquished their licenses because they could not comply with the new standards. Among the laudable innovations the government demands of nursing homes, in addition to new safety regulations, is that more attention be paid to the rehabilitation of the aged, that occupational therapy be instituted, and that social services keep up the families' contact with the residents.

In some well-run nursing homes, the residents participate actively in volunteer services to other aged people, as has been mentioned. This is possible because some larger homes are now located in the center of town and therefore are more accessible for residents' excursions into the world, as well as for visits to them by the family and friends.

Financial Aspects. Unfortunately, it costs a great deal of money to maintain an aged person in a private nursing home. If a lengthy stay is necessary and Medicare payments have run out, the family faces a serious financial drain. The spouse, but not the children, is under obligation to shoulder the financial responsibility for the person in the home. In the end, the resident must spend all his savings until he is reduced to the small sum he is permitted to retain—$1500 for an individual, $2500 for a couple—and can then get Medicaid. He must in effect allow himself to become a pauper. By the time of his death, the spouse may have become a pauper too. This is one of the saddest situations to confront an aged person who has worked hard all his life, who has met all his obligations, and who has been proud that he has not depended on outside help for his health or sustenance. Now that he is old and sick, he must turn to the Welfare Department in order to live.

In analyzing the duration of time an individual spends in a nursing home and his source of support, Dr. Florence Kavaler, then Assistant Commissioner of Health and Medical and Insurance Programs of New York City, Dr. Lowell E. Bellin, present Commissioner of Health, and others, compiled the following figures: 54 per cent stay one year or longer; 21 per cent stay one to two years; 16 per cent stay two to three years; 17 per cent stay three years or longer. They also found that 90 per cent of the residents are supported by Medicaid; 9 per cent pay their own way; and 1 per cent are sponsored by Medicare, which means that the length of stay is limited.*

* Florence Kavaler, Perry G. Haber, and Lowell Eliezer Bellin, "Proprietary Nursing Homes in New York City," *Bulletin of the New York Academy of Medicine*, vol. 49, no. 9 (September 1973), 799.

The striking factor is that only 9 per cent are able to meet the cost of prolonged care from their own funds. At the present time the cost of maintaining a patient in a proprietary nursing home ranges between $1000 and $2000 a month. More than half of nursing-home patients stay a year or longer; clearly a middle-income family can hardly afford this expense. A two- or three-year stay is financially ruinous. These data were gathered in New York City, but the situation is very much the same in every large metropolitan community. It is evident from these figures that a thorough overhaul of public and health insurance in relation to medical and hospital costs is overdue. It should be on the priority list of every public-minded citizen.

One bright spot in the outlook for the future is the continuous growth of geriatric centers that provide services for the aged in their community. It has been found, for instance, that mildly senile old people do not need to be institutionalized as they used to be, but can manage to live by themselves in their accustomed environment as long as the special service of the nearby geriatric center keeps in touch with them regularly, learning about the family relationships, inducing the members of the family to visit the old one oftener, and also arranging for individual and family psychotherapy. In this way, the two generations can be brought together on neutral ground, where they can air their grievances and where they can get to know each other better.

All this makes it obvious that there is a lot of good will but as yet very little action. There is a great deal of confusion about the right way to handle and assist the aged. In an attempt to bring order and clarity into this situation, a group of scientists under the leadership of Dr. T. F. Williams carried out a survey that indicated that a great many of the aged are overevaluated as far as their needs for assistance and care are concerned—a fact that is not constructive and not good for the morale of the patient. They proposed the establishment of a "comprehensive evaluation and

placement service for the ill and the aged." This service would consist of a complete medical and social assessment of the aged person.
In consultation with the family, a recommendation would be made
about where the patient should be placed and what kind of care
would benefit him most. The choices offered are: nursing home,
health-related facility, supervised boarding home, patient's private
home, or psychiatric hospital. Dr. Williams' group believes that
such a service "can achieve significant improvements of elderly
and chronically ill people for long-term care. It can increase an
old one's period of independence and satisfaction. An additional
advantage is the potential savings for the affected persons and the
community through less use of expensive facilities."*

This service is only a beginning, and it will take considerable
time until its utility has been proved, and if so, it will take more
time before it can be applied on an appreciable scale. Meanwhile,
many old people will require assistance and placement in a nursing
home. As I have mentioned several times in other connections, the
federal Department of Health, Education, and Welfare is an excellent source of information, but it is insufficiently known and not
easily accessible to the general public. I would like to draw the
reader's attention to a small pamphlet called *Nursing Home Care,*
Consumer Information Series No. 2, Social and Rehabilitation
Service (SRS) 73-24902. Published in 1973, it is available by
mail from HEW in Washington. In addition to explaining the
various types of nursing homes and their connection with Medicare
and Medicaid, it gives a detailed checklist of what to look for in
a home, which kind of home to select, and which one to avoid, and
similar criteria about the quality of service offered to the prospective resident.

According to community service reports from all over the

* T. F. Williams, J. G. Hill, M. E. Fairbanks, and K. G. Knox, "Appropriate
Placement of the Chronically Ill and Aged," *Journal of the American Medical
Association,* vol. 226, no. 11 (December 1973).

country, more attention should be paid by the public and the authorities to the experimental programs for the study and improvement of the social and economic situation of the aged. It is here that the aged themselves have an almost unplowed and unlimited field for activity since they would be fighting for their own rights and those of future generations. It would also be of immeasurable help if the near-aged also made this struggle for the aged their own.

Twelve

PUTTING THE HOUSE IN ORDER

$\mathcal{T}$he aversion of a great many old people to making a will or revising an outdated one has the same root as the reluctance of most people of all ages to speculate about death. It is much easier for a younger person to make a will, because the prospect of death is so remote that the will is virtually only a gesture, done mostly to please a spouse. But when the end seems to come nearer, making a will is seen as almost the equivalent of signing one's own death warrant. Yet the same person who procrastinates about a will as long as possible will be very conscientious about putting his house in order before he takes a trip. It must be conceded that people of means—especially those who have acquired their wealth themselves—are less hesitant to set down their last dispositions because they feel that they can thereby run things in their own way even from beyond the grave. Moreover, they are under greater pressure from their family than are people who have little to leave behind.

No matter what the circumstances, it is not advisable to make a will without the help of a lawyer. Anyone who is interested in finding out more can write to the Administration on Aging, Department of Health, Education, and Welfare, Washington, D.C., and asking for a booklet called *You, the Law, and Retirement,* by Virginia Lehman (U.S. Government Printing Office, 1972, 0-469-568).

ARRANGING YOUR OWN FUTURE

A person who has made provision for discharging his legal and moral responsibilities has put his house in order only partially. A much more important problem to deal with is what measures to take for his own future in case he becomes physically or mentally unable to manage his own affairs. This is particularly important for an old person who has no close family ties. If he plans to join forces with a friend or a relative, the conditions for the partnership should be clearly defined and put in writing without sentimentality. An old person's memory is not so good as it used to be, and younger people sometimes also suffer from distortions of memory, especially if they are in the wrong and do not want to admit it. It is best if these arrangements are made while the old one is still able to reason things out for himself; otherwise, the aid of an intermediary or a lawyer might be useful.

It is quite possible, however, that a person may be able to live in the community and still need protection for his property and his person because of his disability.* Incapacity to manage one's own affairs may be caused by mental decline, but it may also result from impairment of mobility due to physical illness or weakness. While a person in this condition can be placed under guardianship, and have his property as well as his person cared for, the paradox is that there is no protection that extends to the person only. The reason for this seeming absurdity is that the appointed guardian is entitled to compensation drawn from the estate of the protected one. A person without an estate, or whose estate has been exhausted, is unprotected just at the period of his life when he needs help most.

* This possibility has been ably described by John J. Regan, "Protective Services for the Elderly: Commitment, Guardianship and Alternatives," *William and Mary Law Review*, vol. 13, no. 3 (Spring 1972).

HOW THE GOVERNMENT SHOULD HELP

Here it becomes apparent that outside assistance is needed for two reasons. We are already acquainted with one: after any assets of the protected person have been used up and if he is completely disabled, Medicaid will take over and place him in a nursing home—unless he has been accepted by a subsidized old people's home. In the latter case, the institution acts as his guardian; it will take good care of him and try to rehabilitate him or at least ameliorate his lot. If he is placed in a proprietary nursing home, the money the government provides for his support is—in the absence of a close friend or legal guardian—managed by the nursing-home owner, the very person to whose care the incapacitated person has been entrusted. This impresses me as a clear case of conflict of interest. Since the owner is a businessman who wants and is entitled to make as much profit as possible, how can he be expected to consider the interest of the patient before his own? Some even withhold from the patients the $28 allotted monthly by Medicaid for spending money. There may be a few exceptional owners, but they are certainly not the rule.

The second situation concerns those persons who are mentally enfeebled by age. Not all those so afflicted have to be hospitalized; some can continue living in their usual environment more contentedly than anywhere else, but they need someone to look after them regularly and give assistance where necessary. A striking example of this shook the peace of mind of many concerned citizens when the papers reported a day or two before Christmas 1973 the tragic and needless death of an upstate New York couple in their own home. They were about ninety years old, long out of touch with the world, and having forgotten the modern ways of life, they did not concern themselves about their unpaid bills for gas and electricity. They had the money to pay them but no longer the mentality to act logically. Several well-meaning neighbors and relatives sporadically looked in on them and settled their utility bills, but no one was specifically charged with the duty of looking after their welfare. After the couple was some months in arrears, the utilities cut off service, and the couple then froze to death. Even if they had refused to move to more protected quarters (as was reported), the state has the power to enforce such a move if it is essential to save the lives of the people in question. A consultation with the family might have been sufficient for the life-saving move to have been authorized.

Recently some voices have been raised on behalf of people in similar circumstances. In New York City, the Community Service Society (CSS) has been an ardent proponent of the institution of conservatorship, a service that would look after old people who are "not psychotic but who are temporarily or, in some cases, sporadically incapable of managing their own affairs."* Because of the CSS prodding, the New York State Legislature enacted this proposal into law—but failed to implement it, as has been the case with many other acts to help the aged. Implementation was supposed to be provided in 1973, but as the year ended, nothing had been done. No funds were allotted to run this agency, although it would be easy, as a beginning, to entrust its operations to the highly respected CSS. But there was also no provision for selecting and training the personnel to carry out this long-overdue protection service.

As long as a disabled oldster is in full possession of his faculties he can fight for himself. But should he become forgetful and have difficulty doing simple arithmetic, he is at the mercy of the person who is paid to take care of him unless he has a family or a friend of long standing, or a lawyer whom he has known for a good many years, to check up on things. If he is fortunate enough

* *Bulletin,* Community Service Society of New York, no. 721 (January 1973).

to have maintained old ties that are reliable and not self-seeking, everything is well for the oldster. But if he has lived by himself until old age he may no longer have sufficient judgment to determine the trustworthiness of the person whom he selects to look after him and his interests. One point needs stressing: an old person may be aware of his fading memory, but he will never realize if and when he becomes senile. The simplest illustration of this unawareness is the example of some contemporaries who tell us the same story three or four times during a single lunch, without being conscious of their repetitiveness. If such lapses occur often, they are signs that the mind does not work as well as it used to and may slip back even further.

As some people grow older, they become suspicious of everybody they do not know very well, while others in their loneliness fall for flattery and soft-soaping. Some find new "friends" who are willing to take an old person into their home and promise to look after him as they would for a parent—provided that he makes them his heirs. The oldster is led to believe that he has now found a family, and at first everything goes very well. But if the oldster should live longer than his "foster family" anticipated, his happiness as well as his life may be in danger. In another instance, an oldster takes in an attendant, and after a few months, they become rather friendly, and the attendant suggests that a joint bank account would facilitate dealing with the household expenditures. Once that is done, the attendant disappears with the whole bank account. Confidence men prey by preference on the aged, exploiting their loneliness and need for friends.

ANOTHER SERVICE—FIND

There are several agencies established by the Department of Health, Education, and Welfare, as well as by private social organizations, that try to assist the aged. But they are so little publicized that the ordinary old person or even the ordinary lay person would not know how to locate them and how to enlist their services. Recognizing this, HEW initiated an organization called FIND (for Friendless, Isolated, Needy and Disabled). Although FIND was funded by the Office of Economic Opportunity for the purpose of "exploring the problems of older people in rural areas," the New York City branch carried out an operation in the Times Square area to rescue a number of evicted tenants—the majority of whom were over sixty years old—who were not able to find new lodgings they could afford. Somehow, somewhere, FIND found them adequate inexpensive quarters. With the present governmental economy measures and the current confusion in this field of activity in Washington, it is not certain that this valuable service still exists.

SHOULD A PERSON BE TOLD?

In the last stages of our life, each of us aged people must still face two major problems in the near or relatively near future. One is whether an old person who has only a very short time to live should be told the truth about his impending death or should be left in ignorance or with false hopes. The second problem, now very much in the public eye and just as controversial as the first one, is whether an aged person who is at the brink of death should be kept alive by every possible means or be allowed to sleep over in peace.

I must preface my attempt to offer my conclusions on the first problem by discussing the fear of death. This is a universal, innate reaction; its motivating force is, in my opinion, identical with the struggle for self-preservation. Man clings to life at all costs and by hook or by crook because not living is inconceivable to him. Death means not being in contact with the familiar and not being able to participate in life. I am aware that this is a very simplified formulation of a most complex question that has occupied the interest and research of the philosophers of all times. We do not even know at exactly what age a child becomes old enough to understand death. We do know that a small child begins to cry when Mother, during play, covers her face.

Scientists agree that the greatest calamity that can befall a child is the separation from the protecting mother-figure. We see something akin to this reaction in old people: dislocation from the familiar surroundings can precipitate excitation and confusion; both these symptoms may disappear upon the return to the old environment. The loss of a spouse can have a similar effect and can be ameliorated only by the company of close family members or friends.

Holding on to the familiar is almost like holding on to life, and in this connection, the continuity of life is maintained by various rituals and customs that were practiced at all times and by all people. David Hendin, in an excellent study called *Death as a Fact of Life* explains that funeral procedures, rituals, and ceremonies connected with burial and mourning are attempts to help the survivors to reorient themselves to the changed situation, to offer solace to the survivors, and to give them a period of time for healing. Modern psychiatry and psychology have recognized the therapeutic effect of these customs and of the mourning process as such.

Today very few people in their later years are completely ignorant of the connection between malignant diseases and their threat to life. Public education has progressed quite far during the past few decades, and the time is past when a physician could not admit to a patient that he suffered from a malignant disease—if the patient wanted to know.

As far as the diagnosis or the prognosis is concerned, should a patient be told the truth? The answer depends on the attitude of the three parties involved: the medical personnel, especially the attending physician; the family; and the patient himself. Each of these groups has its own reaction to illness and death, which will determine whether or not a patient is to learn the truth and in what way it should be conveyed to him. In a hospital, the staff generally is in favor of denial, ostensibly because the emotional upheaval caused by revealing the truth to the family may frighten and upset the patient. Actually, the answer depends on the doctor's image of himself as a physician and his relationship to death and dying; it lies in his emotional response to death of a patient who has come to him for help—irrespective of his knowledge of the hopelessness of the case.

In my function as a psychiatrist, I visit the aged patients in a general ward, giving each one the opportunity to talk about himself and the things he cannot discuss with his family. If he has no family, I am the only one who has the time and takes the time to listen; the nurses are too busy to do so. A private doctor will often caution me not to let his patient suspect the correct diagnosis. Having been left in ignorance about the nature of his illness, the patient is sometimes angry with his doctor for not helping him to get better. Some doctors prefer to listen to these reproaches instead of leading the patient gently to learn the truth. And it is an old truism that knowing the facts, however bad, is for some people much less unnerving than perpetual uncertainty.

As far as the family is concerned, the doctor is required by law to inform the next of kin about the true state of affairs. Frequently, it is the family who cannot take the truth or cannot face the patient if he does learn the truth. In some families, it is the custom to be silent about any disagreeable fact, as if it does not exist. These are the families whose members do not communicate with one another although they live under the same roof. To show emotion is embarrassing—it is often considered uncivilized— and to remain hopeful in a crisis helps to hide real feelings. In the case of a fatal illness, the pent-up emotions of the various family members create tension, while the patient is deprived of his right to give vent to his feelings, to his anxieties, and he is also deprived of his right to be solaced. The patient is usually not so ignorant about his state of health as those around him would like to believe. I am convinced that people know in their unconscious when they are fatally ill, in spite of the fact that they may pretend ignorance in order to reassure their family or even themselves. The right time to give a patient the facts of the diagnosis and prognosis authoritatively is when he asks directly or has hinted at it several times. The experienced physician will know whether the patient is ready to hear the truth or whether he is simply looking for "confirmation" that nothing serious is the matter with him.

After they have been told the truth, most patients are grateful for the opportunity to talk about their future and that of their kin. Quite a few grown children have remained their parents' responsibility, although their parents were too proud to admit it and never asked anyone for assistance.

If a person has responsibilities for dependent members of his family or is involved in business transactions that might become muddled in case of his sudden demise, it is the duty of the physician—and no one else—to inform the patient of the nature of his disease so that he can make all provisions necessary to diminish the burdens on the family he is leaving behind. Even if this information would shock the patient at first, he will eventually be most grateful for having been given the opportunity to put his house in order in time. This pertains not only to old people but to people of all ages who suffer from an illness that must end in death. In the case of aged people who have responsibility to a spouse or a middle-aged child who is handicapped in such a way that he will neither be self-supporting nor of assistance to the surviving parent, it is imperative to know the truth.

Some old people, however, will adamantly insist that nothing serious is the matter with them. However, their denial does not necessarily mean that they are ignorant of the true state of affairs; it can mean denial of the truth, which was the case with an eighty-year-old man who was brought to the hospital because of pain in the right side of his chest. Tests showed that he was suffering from lung cancer that had progressed too far for surgical intervention. He gave his family history readily; he mentioned the various relatives—including his own daughter—who had died of lung cancer. He never complained about himself, was always very polite, a model patient. When I invited him to talk about himself, he pointed to the patient in the next bed, commiserating over his illness and emphasizing that this patient was considerably younger than he and yet extremely ill. After he repeated the same maneuver on two other occasions, I stopped trying to make him talk about himself. I was convinced that he knew what was wrong with him but simply did not want to talk about it.

Not everyone bears his unhappiness in silence. I recall a seventy-nine-year-old man who was greatly debilitated by a terminal disease. While clamoring that he wanted to die, he was at the same time seeking as much help as he could get to stem his disease. Since he did not suffer any real pain, it is quite natural that he should want to live, but an observer is quite likely to be taken aback by such contradictory behavior.

While many a young person may rail against being deprived by illness or accident of many years of life, one hears such sentiments very rarely from the aged. After all, people in their seventies and over live on borrowed time, and they know it. I have met only one woman past seventy who cried out when she learned that she was fatally ill: "I am too young to die!"

On the whole, old people do not talk about death or dying among themselves, and it is difficult to get at their real thoughts about it. The healthy aged go about their business as usual, which is a form of denial, but a wholesome one. Others are often seen in their doctor's office hoping to "nip in the bud" the slight ache that may indicate that their end is coming nearer. On the other hand, some withdraw to their quarters, refuse to see a doctor when they are ill, taking a "what's the use" attitude, and are almost scornful of contemporaries who are still active. After having been atheists all their lives, some rediscover religion and derive solace from it now. Still others who fear death more than anything else nevertheless follow the death notices in the newspapers in a self-torturing manner, as if the shrinking of their circle of friends were not enough of a reminder that their own time to die is not far off.

It really cannot be foretold what an old person will do and how he will behave when he realizes that the end is near. Some talk as if they are fully ready to go when their time comes, but still act differently in the end. I remember a woman of eighty who was admitted to the hospital with a spreading malignancy. For the previous fifteen years she had lived with a colostomy and must, therefore, have known the nature of her illness. However, she belonged to a religious sect that denied death, and she explained repeatedly that "dying is just another form of living, because life is eternal." Growing weaker by the day, she reiterated the tenets of her creed over and over again, giving the impression that she was reconciled with what was ahead of her. On the window sill next to her bed stood a small plant some visitor had brought her. When I admired it, she replied that she intended to take the plant home with her after her discharge. Obviously this patient had recited her lessons for many years without conviction and was not prepared to die, despite what she had proclaimed. Eventually she died peacefully in her sleep.

There are signs that old people keep the idea of their impending absence from this world in their minds most of the time. In an almost friendly fashion, an oldster will muse about which one of his or her friends or relatives would enjoy and appreciate a particular trinket that has been dear to him, and now and then he gives away some of these most cherished and most personal items "so that my things will have a home and not be thrown away into the ash can after everything is over."

"DEATH WITH DIGNITY"

I believe that there comes a time in the life of very old people when the fear of death loses a great deal of its terror and is replaced by the fear of pain. I know that several of my contemporaries have accumulated an amount of sedatives sufficient to end their suffering forever if there should be no sympathetic physician around to help them over their last hurdle. The suicide rate among the aged is the highest of all age groups; intractable pain, loneliness, and helplessness rank as the most frequent motivations.

This concept brings us to the second of the problems I mentioned that old people must face—and a topic of heated controversy among thoughtful people: "the right to die with dignity."

The concept of death itself or, better, the absence of life is at present a major subject of medical research and re-evaluation. Up to the present time, a person was pronounced dead when he lost consciousness, had no breath, and his heart stopped beating. The newest research postulates that brain death antecedes the stoppage of the heart. By brain death, we mean that a person is pronounced dead when his brain ceases to respond to electric stimulation; his heart can be kept beating by artificial means even after the brain stops reacting to the electric stimulation.

These findings demand re-evaluation of the methods currently applied to the concept of preserving or saving life. It must be stated emphatically that every person has the right to die peacefully and in dignity.

While any available method should be utilized to keep a young person alive, or an old one who has a chance of returning to at least a tolerable existence, this should not apply to people who do not have this chance, especially those whose death is imminent for reasons other than the occurrence that brought them to the brink of death. In other words, a person who is dying has the right to pass away without having to undergo the ordeal of being kept alive artificially on principle. He has the right to be made as free from suffering as possible for the time that is left to him, but there should be no prolongation of life for its own sake. For instance, a person who is dying of a malignancy that has progressed so far as to make his death imminent in a day or two should not be given a blood transfusion just to make him live longer.

I hope, when my time comes, that no one will try to keep me going with any kind of medication or apparatus. All I expect is to be made comfortable, since I do not like pain. I have instructed my doctor, my lawyer, and my friends to comply with that wish.

Some countries have certain provisions to assist suffering people in their last days or hours—an idea very different in principle from the concept of euthanasia that was propounded during the 1920s. This humane idea fell into disrepute when it was misused during the Hitler regime to rid Germany of nonproductive citizens (leaving fewer mouths to feed). According to David Hendin, Switzerland has a law that allows a physician to hand his dying patient a lethal dose of a sedative, but the doctor is not permitted to administer it himself. This gives the patient a choice and expresses his right as an individual to do with his life as he pleases.

A similar principle was at work in the following instance that was reported in the October 1973 issue of *New York Medicine*, the official organ of the New York County Medical Association. An elderly woman suffering from a terminal disease that caused her great pain refused to accept treatment that would have prolonged her life for a short time. The general hospital in Palm Springs, Florida, where the patient was being cared for, took the case to court because time and again, a court order has been obtained holding that life-saving treatment may be applied even if the patient or his relatives do not consent. In this case, however, the court held that "In these circumstances any conscious adult had the right to refuse treatment."

There is, however, another group of aged people who are just as deserving of being liberated from unbearable suffering but who are unable to exercise the privilege of decision because they are mentally incapable of doing so; their minds have deteriorated through age or through a fatal illness so that they have lost touch with the world entirely. Medical science knows that these changes due to age are irreversible. Why should a person who has become so mentally incapacitated that he does not recognize his nearest relative, and has to be fed artificially, receive a heart stimulus if he suffers a heart attack? I believe it would be kinder to keep him peaceful and comfortable rather than to try to rescue the function of his heart. He is an individual who has no livable world to come back to.

LEGAL AND RELIGIOUS CONSIDERATIONS

Much public education is needed before it will be possible to protect this "right to die with dignity" through legislation. Legislation concerning this is being introduced in some states, and I am sure there will be more to come. Proper safeguards can be established to prevent misuse and to reassure the family that no error occurred.

Since the people most interested in it are the aged, it is up to them to raise their voices and fight for this right—and others.

There may be objections on moral and religious grounds, although the humane elements cannot be denied. It may ease the mind of people who are not sure whether their religious creed would sanction a policy of this kind to learn that neither the Catholic nor the Jewish religion is against it. Let me quote from a paper by Dr. Joseph G. Zimring: "The law should recognize that a physician with or without relatives' permission, can discontinue extraordinary means of sustaining life when clinical death is inevitable and when there is no possibility of recovery." Dr. Zimring strengthens his argument with these two quotations: "Pope Pius XII in 1957 stated: 'Human life continues for as long as its vital functions, distinguished from the simple or biologic life of the organs, manifest themselves spontaneously without the help of artificial processes. . . . The task of determining the exact instant of death is that of the physician.' "* The second quotation is from "the Halacha, laws found in the Talmud, [which] states: 'We are forbidden to shorten the life of a dying man by even one moment. But it is also forbidden to prolong his life artificially when there are no prospects for him to remain alive.' "

These two statements speak for themselves and should help in bringing acceptance of the humanity of the new concept.

IMMORTALITY?

Recently a man in his late sixties asked me what I thought about life after death. This same question has been put to me many

---

* "The Right to Die with Dignity," *New York State Journal of Medicine*, July, 1973. Dr. Zimring wrote in his capacity as chairman of the Committee on Ethics and assistant secretary of the Medical Society of the State of New York and director of family practice at Long Beach Memorial Hospital, New York.

times by old people and young ones whom I counseled or in an ordinary conversation. Since time immemorial philosophers have devoted themselves to the penetration of this mystery, without results. Religion, too, has been occupied with this problem, and each denomination has its own theory. It has been my custom to refer those who asked me this question to the representatives of their church, but sometimes they insist on knowing what I personally think about it.

I am no philosopher, but I believe that there is no thoughtful person who has not pondered this idea in one way or another. I also believe that everyone has a solution worked out according to his own private philosophy.

I believe that every human being is actually immortal, but not quite in the sense in which that word is generally used. My idea is that in your contact with people, good and bad, an image of you is created in the other person; for instance, a resident in the institute where I teach learns from me some things he finds useful and is going to apply in his later work. The same immortality has been accorded by me to my teachers, when I quote them to my students. If I apply this kind of "living on" to my former patients and to some of my friends with whom I exchanged opinions and whose worries and joys I shared, just as they did mine, then I continue living in each of them even if they eventually forget that I ever existed.

Immortality becomes more tangible with people who have children. Their chromosomes and genes, which they inherited from their parents, are transmitted to their offspring. And the sense of values a child develops is part of his mother's and father's conscience; this too represents the continuity that we may call immortality.

As long as I am able to conceive life and its end in this fashion, fear of death seems to recede into the background. I am aware of the fact that anything good or bad one did to people has the same self-perpetuating effect. All that anyone who has filled his place in this world can hope for is that the positive influences he has had on people will outweigh the negative. Since I do not believe in any reward in another world, I am, by the same token, not afraid of punishment. It would sound sanctimonious if I said that I tried the best I could. I can only say I lived as decently as I could.

Thirteen

THE SUMMING UP

$\mathscr{W}$hen I came to summarize my findings, I realized how much I had not known when I began this study and how many unanswered questions still remained. There was one specific question I had often asked myself and as many other old people as I could buttonhole: "When did you feel you were getting old?" I found that the answers fell into three main categories. The most frequent reply was: "I do not feel old. I feel the same as I always did." The second group referred to a specific event in the person's external life, such as: "When my husband retired," "When my wife died," "When I acquired a daughter-in-law," "When my youngest child got married," or "When I became a grandmother." In the third group, the blame was put on the onset of diseases that occur most often in, but are not confined to, later years. Such illnesses as arthritis or high blood pressure cause a great deal of discomfort and often restrict their victim's activity and, therefore, are readily made scapegoats.

Since it cannot be denied that aging is a progressive process that inescapably takes its toll, one learns upon continuous questioning that the aged, especially those who are in full command of their faculties, are aware of their diminishing physical prowess, of some impairment of the sense organs, and of occasional lapses of memory. These lessenings of function come on so imperceptibly that they are integrated into the daily life without the aging person's admitting, even to himself, that the change in his mode of living is actually due to getting older. When I put my question to an elderly self-employed businessman, he denied at first that he felt his age, but as we continued talking, he mentioned with a kind of sheepish grin that he had recently placed a couch in his office so that he could take a rest between clients.

Apart from the mechanism of denial, with which we are already acquainted, there are other reasons for the seeming failure to perceive change in the course of years. Sometimes there is an unintended falsification of memory caused by wishful thinking, as this anecdote illustrates: after a recent snowfall, a contemporary of mine mentioned how beautiful the fresh snow appeared as she looked out of her window. She added how glad she was, at the same time, that she did not have to go out that day and face the snow. Suddenly she remembered that in her youth and even much later she could not wait on a snowy day until she could get out and romp around in it. She is one of those people who has always maintained that she does not feel any different now from the way she did when she was young. She has tried very hard, as so many other old people do, to hold on to a self-image from the past that does not correspond to the facts of her present situation.

I must clarify one point now. The near-aged and the aged are quite justified in denying that they feel their age. They remain much younger, much healthier, and more active than our parents and grandparents did. It is the people seventy-five and over who begin to feel their age and still try desperately to hang on to the denial with all their might and to retain recollections of former days to persuade themselves that they could be young, if they tried hard enough. One fact is certain and cannot be stressed strongly enough. No matter what his age, as long as a person lives, he has feelings, desires, and needs that are no different from those he had when young. To feel pushed aside as useless and super-fluous is just as painful at eighty as it is at twenty. This is what the younger generation cannot understand. *Emotions in a mentally alert older person may be less intense as the years go by, but they exist and are inseparable from living.* It will take a great deal of education of the aged themselves, and of the younger generation, before they will accept this unalterable connection between all ages.

Because of this universality of human reaction, no distinction has been made in this study along ethnic lines. People, no matter of what origin, are people, as Shakespeare observed in the passage quoted in the first chapter. Various subcultures and family struc-tures may differ in small details. It appears that old people who live in a culture that still adheres more or less to the extended fam-ily are somewhat better protected from the vicissitudes of old age and poverty than those who live in the nuclear family setting. How-ever, there seem to be no perceptible differences deriving from disparate religious creeds.

The next question I posed was whether the lot of the aged has improved during the last decade or two. I also wanted to find out about the chances for further improvements. Two main cate-gories are pertinent in interpreting my findings: one is the eco-nomic situation of the aged after retirement and their resultant standard of living; the other is the education of younger people in understanding the aged, and subsequently, inseparably tied to this fact, is the preparation of the individual for his own old age.

The economic situation of the aged and the improvement of their standard of living depends largely on government legislation and on the development of a fair and healthy pension system. The new regulations that automatically would link Social Security benefits to the cost of living index, together with the creation of the "portable" pension plan advocated by Senator Philip Hart of Michigan and the proposals laid down by Ralph Nader in *You and*

Your Pension offer a genuinely constructive start in the right direction. The first proposal would remove Social Security payments from politics, and the second would assure the worker that the money he and his employer contribute to the eventual pension will actually be used for the worker's benefit.

Up to the present, whenever economic retrenchment has been in order, budgetary cuts usually have begun with that group that is expendable because it is nonproductive—namely, the aged. It is up to them, to their fighting spirit and their ability to acquire allies among the younger people, if a stop is to be put to slashing government expenditures among the neediest because they are the most helpless group. The public conscience must be mobilized.

PREPARATION FOR OLD AGE—IS IT POSSIBLE?

During the last decades people have been living longer because the degenerative diseases have become more and more amenable to treatment. Even though not all of them can be cured or prevented as yet, the increasing ability to control pain diminishes the wear and tear on the energies of the afflicted person, a fact that may influence the lengthening of man's span of life. Scientists, however, are not certain that curing these diseases will actually prolong the life of everybody.

As Lewis Thomas explains, man, like everything else in nature, is programed to die after a predetermined length of time clocked by his genomes (chromosomes). "If this is the way it is, some of us will continue to wear out and come unhinged in the sixth decade, and some much later, depending on genetic timetables."*

* Lewis Thomas, *The Lives of a Cell* (New York: The Viking Press, 1974). Dr. Thomas, a former dean at Yale Medical School, serves as president of the Memorial Sloan-Kettering Cancer Center in New York.

Other geneticists have expressed similar views: that the life span of an individual is determined by his heredity in the same way as are the color of his eyes, his height, and other characteristics that "run in families." Even if we cannot expect to match eventually the years Methusaleh and other biblical fathers were supposed to have reached, we can assume that more and more people will reach ripe old age in the future.

This outlook is a most appealing one because old people's energies will be increasingly liberated for useful and more satisfying forms of living. It may take more time to accomplish this than we oldsters have at our disposal, but it is a pleasure to anticipate that our successors will reap the benefits of our efforts, our labors, and our sacrifices.

This new vista of the future of the elderly creates new needs for a proper preparation for being old. As Sidney P. Marland, Jr., has stated: "At a time when life expectancy is moving into the seventies, the notion that a person should be trained for a single vocation is obsolete."* I fully agree with this statement; in the chapter on the use of leisure, I have shown the advantages of a broadly based general education and the possibilities it affords for various occupational choices in later life.

The idea of preparing for more than one career has long been adopted by people whose work demanded a great deal of physical exertion and who therefore have a limited period of maximum efficiency—for instance, professional athletes follow a trade at the same time as they train for their athletic competitions. Some become coaches or teach their specialty after their prime years have passed. The same is true for performing artists for whom appearance is at a premium.

---

* "Education for More than One Career," *World*, July 18, 1972. Dr. Marland was at that time U.S. Commissioner of Education.

Men and women in government service, such as military personnel, firemen, and policemen, who may retire on half pay after twenty years of service, have also pursued more than one career. They have usually entered private employment in a capacity similar to their former activity. Recently, however, they have been seeking more education—going to law school or into the public-health field. A case in point: early in 1973, eighty-four men and women who had retired from public service in various New York City departments graduated as registered nurses after going to night school in a special program given by the Hunter College School of Nursing during the last two and a half years of their municipal service. After working for the city for at least twenty years, these men and women have sufficient retirement pay to cushion their future, and, in their second career, they will be able to work longer with less strain on their physical energies than in their previous posts. Others have taken similar paths: specialists such as engineers and lawyers have added education in management and are utilizing their double training to their own and their employers' advantage. Similarly, men and women working on assembly lines fought for and won assignments to a rotating schedule of tasks in order to be relieved of the monotony of their work and to acquire broader training.

The same trend can be seen among women in their forties and older who return to the labor force as soon as their children no longer need day-long attention. Some resume the kind of work they were originally trained for, but a surprising number take a different path. Often the new calling they choose is working with handicapped children, especially brain-damaged ones. No special schooling is needed for this work, only patience and love for children. The pay is low, but the reward is high—it is the affection these rejected children bestow so liberally on those who protect and look after them.

Preparation for old age includes more than learning a second trade or changing one's job around retirement time. It also means rearranging our lives so that we do not inflict irreparable damage to one organ system or another by misuse or abuse. I strongly suspect that the extraordinary stress put on athletic prowess in the early years contributes greatly to the large number of damaged hearts in relatively young persons. By the same token, the lack of proper food is known to create havoc with the aged who are poor. But it is not only poverty that is responsible for malnutrition, with all its consequences, but also wrong food habits, unnecessary diets and food fads, etc., in the younger years. We should also learn to eradicate pollution in the air we breathe, the food we eat, and the water we drink; they all influence our body chemistry and eventually our bodily functions.

THE OUTLOOK FOR THE FUTURE

It is not only the physical condition of our environment that will influence the degree to which the last portion of our lives can be lived and enjoyed. The numerous social changes under way at present may have considerable influence on our future modes of living. Two tendencies in particular whose outcome cannot be foreseen involve the aged. One is the effect the inevitable advent of the four-day work week will have on the labor market for the aged; the other is the changing relationship between the sexes.

Because of the first, younger workers may begin to compete for the part-time jobs retired aged workers currently fill. The second trend may have a profound impact on the living arrangements of the aged. Until a short time ago, division of labor between the male and the female was rather sharply drawn: women worked in and around the house and took care of the children and the sick, while men "brought home the bacon" and defended the family and their people in general against enemies from outside. I call this a longitudinal division of labor, in which male and female complemented each other, and their well-defined functions left no doubt in the minds of their children about the sex of each parent, as well as their own. In emergencies, the roles were at times temporarily reversed. Gradually, the emancipation of women began to make inroads into the masculine world, although women rarely gained first-rank positions. When men were doing women's work, they were the exception, and they covered up this "degradation" with an exalted title. A woman who prepared food was a cook, while a man who did the same was a chef. A woman who sewed for a living was a seamstress, while her male counterpart was a tailor, etc., etc.

This longitudinal division is in the process of becoming a horizontal one. As instruments and tools were invented that substituted for physical strength, more and more women have begun to do men's work, while quite a few men are entering women's fields. In other words, the complementation is giving way to competition. In addition, up to now mankind procreated through the union of the two sexes, however temporary such a union may have been. Since artificial insemination can make a woman pregnant, she can actually dispense entirely with personal contact with the male if she wishes. Whether this is of advantage to her depends on the nature of her personality. It certainly will be of no advantage to the offspring, be it a boy or a girl, and the "independent" woman may realize years later what injustice and emotional damage she inflicted on her child.

If this trend continues, the structure of the family may be narrowed even more than it already has been. This would undoubtedly have an effect on the place the aged would have in the new society. The impact of this trend on the younger and even the older generation is already noticeable in some respects. The new kinds of family the younger generation is experimenting with—group marriage or "marriage" with a member of the same sex—makes it even less inviting for an old parent to seek a haven in his child's home or even near it. It is equally difficult to move in with a child's family in which the wife goes to work and the husband takes care of the household chores on a permanent basis. If the husband should be unable to go to work because of illness, and his wife must seek employment to help with the family income, the presence of an aged parent who can still lend a hand may be very welcome. But when the parent becomes feeble and in need of assistance, living in a household in which the roles are permanently reversed may not be to his liking, or to his children's.

This new arrangement in a younger couple's marriage is fundamentally different from the one where the aged husband takes over the household chores because his wife is sick and unable to function or because—as discussed earlier in this book—she still goes to work while he has already retired. In such cases, the husband does not give it a second thought when he prepares the meals and enjoys doing so. There is no thought that he might be called a sissy because he is doing women's work—and likes it.

But for younger couples to reverse the roles of male and female is bound to reflect on their respect and devotion for each other and does not provide good auspices for the permanency of their marriage. It is to be hoped that these experimentations will remain just that, and that in time the family will be restored to its biological function as the basis for men and women to live together.

These reflections lead me rather far afield from the original topic of evaluating whether the lives of the aged are easier today than in the past. But these social mutations do play a part, and no one can foretell what effect they will have on life in old age.

PUBLIC AWARENESS

Amid all these uncertainties there are still a good many encouraging signs that the public is becoming aware of the justified needs of the older age groups. In the fall of 1971, the White House Conference on Aging was held in Washington. It would go beyond the scope of this study to go into detail about this conference.* However, I do want to say that I was deeply impressed with the participants' insight, sympathy, and ingenuity in planning remedies. Whether all the ideas can ever be put into practice is not for me to say, however. Several proposals at this conference are worthy of mention because of their simplicity and their human potentialities. There were recommendations for dispensing information on old age in every school, at every level, from the elementary grades through the colleges and universities. This makes a great deal of sense because, as a result of the change from the extended to the nuclear family, children have little opportunity for close contact with the older generation.

The recommendations that grew out of this conference gave the official stamp of approval to various efforts along similar lines that have been under way for the past few years. One government program within the framework of the HEW agency called ACTION (for: "Actions speak louder than words") is ACE. Though still operating on a small scale, ACE makes it possible for a college student, as part of his educational program, to devote one year with full academic credit to the study of underprivileged minorities, including the aged poor.

Two new specialties dealing with the aged are actually beginning to be taught at colleges as part of the medical, paramedical,

* The final report, *Toward a National Policy on Aging*, can be obtained from the Superintendent of Documents, U.S. Government Printing Office, Washington, D.C. 20402, at $6.75 for the two-volume set.

and sociological programs. One is geriatrics, the branch of medical science that deals with the treatment and research of illnesses usually occurring in old age and with the aging process as such. The other is gerontology, the social counterpart of geriatrics. Gerontology concerns the social, economic, and human aspects of the lives of the aged.

The student concentrating on gerontology will have courses in social work with the aged, housing, recreation, and other services to the aged, such as geriatric nursing and related subjects.

As these projects gain momentum, they will eventually acquaint larger numbers of the young with the special needs of the older generation; they will bring the young and the old together so that both can learn to communicate with one another. Learning about their similarities and differences may be of immediate help to the aged, but for the young it will also be an excellent preparation for their own old age looming at the other end of life.

The report of the Conference on Aging also cites many ways—although they are still small in scale—in which various communities and individuals help to bring some pleasure into the lives of the old. For instance, reduced prices for admission to some movie theaters during the afternoon hours, or to some ball games. Cut-rate transportation on buses and even in taxis in parts of the country without bus service is a valuable boon, for visits have to be made to doctors or to a hospital for regular treatment, or to the houses of worship that are vital to many old people. At least once in a while, they will also want to visit friends and relatives who live too far away to be reached by walking; otherwise the oldsters would be very isolated and feel as if they were in prison if they have no means of leaving the house.

The most encouraging proposals center on the schools: to let the poor aged partake of hot lunches wherever they are provided for school children; to admit oldsters to grade schools together with the children, to learn or to improve their ABCs, or to learn English if they are foreign-born. They need to know the language in order to decide for whom to vote, to read the labels of the food they buy, and to understand what they are signing when they enter into a contract or other agreement.

A beginning has been made in narrowing the gap between the young and the old through the Foster Grandparents project. The popularity of this HEW-sponsored plan speaks for itself, as was noted in Chapter 7. Another project that impresses me as offering even greater significance in bringing the generations together is being tried out in Connecticut. In this program, elderly people are teamed up with "learning disabled" students in the middle schools. *The New York Times* of March 2, 1974, reported that: "Aside from academic tutoring in reading, language development, math and writing the volunteers share their special skill with youngsters interested, say, in electronics. The tutoring is done on a one-to-one basis and the tutor is paid a nominal fee." The advantages are immeasurable for both parties: not only will the student profit, not only will the two generations become better acquainted, but the tutor himself will have the rare opportunity of being needed, being appreciated, and being forced to keep up to date in his own field if he is to be effective as a teacher. Moreover, the pleasure a good teacher feels when he sees a glimmer of understanding in the eyes of his pupils is one of the satisfactions that can almost never be duplicated. Being an old hand at teaching on a one-to-one basis, I can testify to this fact.

SELF-HELP

In spite of these and other programs that have been initiated by the Department of Health, Education, and Welfare, as well as by industry and labor, real help can come only from the aged themselves and from the near-aged, who are next in line, but are still strong and vigorous enough to lead the fight. There are quite a number of organizations of the aged; the largest are listed in Appendix A under the heading "Organizations."

If the aged are to be freed from the universal ostracism that they still experience today, if they are to be freed from the condescension of some of their well-wishers, they should unite under well-known and respected leadership and make themselves heard, seen, and appreciated through their actions and initiatives. There are many elder statesmen or members of Congress or other people who are widely esteemed who would qualify by age and talent to be the leaders. Through a joint effort of this kind, the aged could become people again, instead of being objects no longer usable.

Let us not forget that there are 20 million people sixty-five and over in our country, representing 10 per cent of the total population, a number that increases year by year far more rapidly than the total population. In other words, the relative strength of the aged is large and growing. Politicians and the leaders of various interest groups ought to pay attention to the aged, and the voices of the aged should be listened to with more consideration and sympathy than heretofore—especially since the interests of the aged are not altered by subcultures, political associations, and religious creeds that could be misused for political purposes by playing one group against another. For everybody gets older, no matter where he comes from, and no matter how he votes. Nor is the buying power of such a large group, with no need to make further savings, to be underestimated either.

As this study comes to a close, a reader who has several choices in organizing his life after he is no longer forced to work for his living might want to know my judgment on which of the several paths that have been shown would be the most satisfactory

way to live out his days. It would be folly to attempt to advise anyone whom one does not know personally; even if one does know
the person, the risk of making a mistake would be great. Tastes
and inclinations are as numerous as there are people; each one has
to make his own decisions in this respect.

Yet listening to and observing old people who seem content
and who seem to stay young longer, especially in spirit, even if
their bodies have become frail and tired, one finds one common de-
nominator: the people for whom old age has been most rewarding
are those who are able to share with others the knowledge and the
experience they have accumulated in their lifetime. It is my firm
belief that an old person who has spent his life collecting skills
and wisdom that cannot be learned from books, but must be acquired from life by trial and error, feels that he is in debt to all
the people from whom he has learned and who have enriched his
life and widened his horizon. There is only one way of repaying
this debt; that is, by sharing this stock of experience with others
who may do likewise when their time comes.

I readily concede that only a relatively small group of people
is privileged to do so on a substantial scale, but I would like to
remind the reader of the sharing that is being done in small ways
by all the many elderly volunteers who are squaring the account
I just mentioned by their contributions to their fellow men in their
own way. Whether you have old people helping other elderly ones
with their daily chores or whether there is an oldster who teaches
a small child how to whistle, the result is the same for both parties
—the teacher as well as the pupil, the helper and the one who is
being helped both profit and are made happier, the former because
his life is being made meaningful again, and the latter, old or
young, is reassured that he has not been entirely cast aside by life.

If I should be pressed for more specific suggestions, I would
say, pick a project that you want to pursue, irrespective of the

need for time and irrespective of your chance to see the project through to its end. Unless you have a purpose in life, expressed in its simplest form—"something to get up for in the morning"—you begin to stagnate, and that is the worst thing any old person could or should do. Yet if an old person feels that all he wants to do is sit and rest, he is entitled to do so, because everyone has the right to be happy in his own fashion.

Appendix A

FACILITIES

*T*his section contains a guide to sources of information concerning the major aspects of our lives. The most comprehensive sources are the federal, state, and city offices of our government. There are two main ways to get correct information about almost anything that concerns the individual citizen. You may, of course, inquire directly of these government agencies if you have a specific problem. However, almost every old person can benefit from reading two publications issued specifically for them.

I cannot recommend highly enough the monthly magazine *Aging*, issued by the Department of Health, Education, and Welfare, Office of Human Development, Administration on Aging. To subscribe for a year, send your name and address, accompanied by a check or money order for $4.50, to: The Superintendent of Documents, Washington, D.C. 20402. *Aging* reports on all official measures taken by the federal government and the individual states on behalf of the aged. Newly enacted regulations are listed and new benefits described. Since these vary from state to state, and pertain to many different aspects of our lives, it is difficult to obtain up-to-date information on them. Through *Aging* magazine, every aged person can keep himself informed about what goes on in his state and can, therefore, easily get in touch with the agency that sponsors the innovation or deals with other relevant matters.

Another magazine containing information of interest to the aged is the *Newsletter* issued by the American Association of Retired Persons. This publication is available only to members of this organization. Application for membership, which costs $2.00 per year, should be addressed to the AARP, c/o Postmaster, Washington, D.C. 20006. Be sure to include a request for this *Newsletter*.

While the Department of Health, Education, and Welfare (HEW), Washington, D.C. 20506, is the federal agency concerned with the aged, and it will certainly answer your questions or refer you to some organization that will, I think that it will be preferable —certainly faster and easier—to deal with local agencies.

On the local level, there are HEW branch offices in the larger cities. On the whole, however, the state and city agencies are of greater practical help in giving individuals information as well as advice and assistance. No general instructions can be given on the methods of the various agencies because each has its own system of approach. But no one can fail to get an answer if he writes or telephones the department dealing with his particular question. State agencies are usually located in the state capital; many have branch offices throughout the state. The local authorities in your home town are actually the best bet to try first because they are the most accessible to the advice seeker.

In addition to the government agencies on various levels, there are the many religious and philanthropic organizations (the latter, in many instances, are also organized along denominational lines); and there are large social-service organizations for individuals and families that are geared to give counsel and assist persons in need. Your own church is one of the most natural and promising sources for guidance, not only in religious matters but also in any others that are vital to the individual. Every community, large or small, has religious centers oriented to specific denominations, but to my knowledge, almost none confines itself to its own membership; each is willing to assist anyone who comes for help. In case it is not able to do so, it will certainly refer you to the proper channels.

Social-service organizations, settlement houses, and neighborhood associations are well known to the residents, young or old, whom they serve in the vicinity where they are located. A look in the telephone book or a question to a neighbor or the superintendent of the building you live in will guide you to the proper place. Any day center for older people will gladly refer you to the agency from whom you can expect help.

I have listed below, in alphabetical order, the various categories of services and information important in the lives of the aged.

EDUCATION

If a person wants to finish his elementary schooling up to the eighth grade, he should get in touch with the local board of education. The public schools offer classes on various levels in all the subjects required to enable the student to get a qualifying certificate; he may even earn a high-school diploma. There are also classes in which English is taught to the foreign-born. For these no special requirements need be met, and no tuition is charged. In some smaller communities, it is even possible for aged students to sit in with grade-school children in regular daytime classes.

A person who already has a high-school diploma or its equivalent may apply to a college as a full-time student or go to night school, where the number of courses required is half the number demanded of full-time students; in this way, the oldster may take his time and adjust the tempo of his education to the degree of his energy. He has all the time in the world at his disposal, since nothing seriously depends on his finishing the program.

If he does not have a high-school diploma, the newly established community colleges are open to him; there any student may take as many courses as he is capable of doing justice to without any pressure of time.

In larger communities, there are also a number of adult-education projects, usually connected with institutions of higher learning, where anyone (even without formal education) may attend individual courses in subjects that interest him—just for the pleasure of knowing more about them. At the end of the course, he can usually take an examination and get a certificate stating that he has successfully attended the course. In this way, one may even collect credits at a leisurely pace that may lead to a degree. Most of the courses are given both in the daytime and in the evening.

New York University has extension courses of this kind, and the New School for Social Research has an extensive adult-education program. These are two of the best known facilities in Manhattan, but there are many others elsewhere in the city, and every larger community or suburb has similar institutions. If the prospective student does not know their addresses, or if he wants to locate such a school in a community he plans to move to but where he does not yet know the ropes, there is a simple way to find out: by visiting his local library. Libraries throughout the country are in communication with each other, and if one library in one town needs information of this sort, it can get it—and with pleasure— from a library in another locality.

If the community is too small to house a college or university, the head librarian or the school librarian will be glad to assemble a reading list for home study. It is also possible for older people to form a study group of their own, and I am sure that the principal of the local school would arrange for professional supervision through a member of his staff. This do-it-yourself method can go a long way toward creating a meaningful life and avoiding boredom and mental stagnation.

Arts and crafts are taught under the same sponsorship as academic subjects. They are also taught in day centers for senior citizens as part of the occupational activities for the elderly. The teachers there are often quite well-trained artists who give some of their time as volunteers to the older generation. For the latter there is the added advantage that all the fellow students are contemporaries, and there is a good chance to make a few friends and to find suitable companionship.

In some states there is a new area of assistance to old people who have difficulty getting about. A bookmobile makes the rounds to nursing homes and individual residences every two weeks, with a librarian in attendance who can advise on the selection of reading matter and provide a program for further reading.

How intense and how universal the desire for more knowledge is among the aged of most nations can be gauged from the fact that a university exclusively for the elderly has been established in Toulouse, France, with an enrollment of a thousand students whose average age is seventy.

HEALTH

Every aged person should carry his Medicare identification card on his person, together with the name and telephone number of his personal physician, his blood type (if possible), and the name and telephone number of his next of kin. These data will save a great deal of time and may even save his life if they are readily available.

If you become sick, consult your family doctor. He is connected with a hospital and will be able to obtain a bed for you in case of need and make all other arrangements that are necessary on your behalf. If you want to secure a private physician, the local or county medical society will recommend one through its referral service. Since very few doctors make house calls, especially at night, except to patients they have known for a long time, you might ask the same referral service to supply the names of doctors who do make house calls.

If you cannot get medical aid in an emergency, have a friend accompany you to the emergency room of the nearest hospital. If you cannot make it under your own steam, call the police, who will summon an ambulance for you. Once you are in the hospital, let the authorities there take over. You can request transfer to the hospital of your choice or to the geriatric section, if you are not already in it. When the time for discharge comes, the social-service department of the hospital will assist you to make plans about either returning home or going to an extended-care facility, where you may stay until you are ready to return to your own home. In Chapter 12, I described the various forms of care an old person may avail himself of when sick or too feeble to manage living by himself.

I would like to draw attention to the various rehabilitation centers. You should consult one of them during convalescence if there is a sickness or an accident that may lead to lasting impairment of mobility. It would be to any family's advantage to have an aged member examined and advised by such a center before it places him in a nursing home for the rest of his life.

The various kinds of home-care services, so enthusiastically heralded by the federal agencies as new institutions designed to keep the elderly in their usual environment and at lower cost than in nursing homes, are unfortunately available only on a very limited basis. Many hospitals are not yet geared to such an expansion of their services. There are not as yet enough people trained for the kind of work that is needed in order to be of help to the infirm and sick aged. Moreover, neither Medicare nor Medicaid so far covers homemaker and housekeeper services. It is necessary to rely on volunteer services rendered by neighbors and friends, which are often not sufficient.

HOUSING

Housing is the area where I can be of the least help. Old people who can afford it will find no difficulties if they want to change their living arrangements. The ones who want to follow the sun will have many renting agents on their trail to give them detailed and perhaps somewhat exaggerated information; fortunately quite a few people in times past have visited the places where they would like to live and have made their choices some time before. They may even have friends who moved earlier to the same place, and they, therefore, do not need any direction.

However, for those who need help very badly, there is little to offer at present, and I am afraid this will be the case for some time to come. I am thinking of the middle- and low-income aged with or without families. The shortage of housing, the long waiting lists, and the plight of the single aged poor living under disastrous conditions have often been publicized of late; I do not need to go into detail about them here. Yet it has always been my firm belief that no problem is insoluble. We may not be able to find a solution within a few weeks or months, and we may not be able to give much practical help to the present generation of aged that is exposed to so much degradation. But we can begin solving it by educating the near-aged who are still young enough to fight and to do some lobbying to prod the people in office to pay attention and to act on behalf of the old. Sufficient housing for the aged should be on the priority list of every lawmaker; proper provisions of an economic and a social nature should be established *and* implemented so that the extreme poverty of such a large portion of our aged population can be eradicated. To have the laws on paper is not enough: they must be put into action.

JOBS

Before a worker retires, he usually participates in a series of seminars and consultations, sponsored either by his company or his union, that prepare him for the new life he is about to begin. Included in these sessions is information about what kinds of jobs exist and how to look for them. If the financial situation of a retired person is not too precarious, part-time jobs are preferable because they save energy and also leave some time for play.

State employment agencies with offices in almost every town in the country have listings of available jobs and arrange for testing and counseling without a fee. The federal Office of Economic Opportunity recommends both part-time jobs and volunteer work, and a combination of the two seems to me the most desirable. This means that working time is limited to twenty hours a week, and the pay is the current minimum wage (there are a few jobs that pay slightly more and others that refund out-of-pocket expenses such as transportation and lunches). Detailed information about these jobs can be obtained by writing to the Department of Health, Education, and Welfare, Washington, D.C. 20506. If you live in a large city, there will be a local office whose phone number and address are listed in the telephone directory. It will respond with utmost courtesy to your inquiries.

Philanthropic and religious organizations as well as settlement houses in larger communities are ready to assist any aged person to locate a job, usually a part-time or free-lance one. Some of these organizations also provide free training for these jobs. In addition, there are sheltered workshops, run usually by philanthropic organizations, where aged persons who are slightly handicapped can find work. The operations of some of these workshops were described in the chapter on volunteer work.

LEGAL SERVICES

Anyone who is in need of legal advice and does not have a personal lawyer can get in touch with the local bar association, which maintains a referral service. If the aged person looking for legal advice cannot pay a regular lawyer's fee, he should turn to the local branch of the Legal Aid Society. But remember that anyone who receives public assistance is entitled to free legal representation and advice; details of this service are available through the local HEW office for the aged.

One may wonder what kind of legal problems the aged may have that younger people do not. The FIND project carried out in New York City to aid aged people too helpless and too uninformed to seek assistance due them (see Chapter 12) is ample proof that special problems exist. Some old people are too feeble or too uneducated to follow the newspaper reports of new rulings on their behalf and are incapable of making use of them. They may need help, for instance, with their landlords, some of whom are neglectful in making needed repairs and maintaining the minimum legal temperature or who balk at complying with the laws exempting the aged poor (sixty-two and over) from rent increases in rent-controlled buildings—a fact that some oldsters are unaware of or that they do not know how to utilize. Some of the rulings come in so fast that they are at times contradictory or antiquated before they are put into action. Moreover, some landlords want to get the aged tenants out of their buildings and do their best to make life unpleasant for them.

There are problems with pensions and pension rights, wills have to be made, debts have to be paid as well as collected, and many other instances arise where the oldster cannot manage by himself. There is a federally financed project called Legal Service for the Elderly Poor, 2095 Broadway, New York, N.Y. 10023;

telephone: 595-1340. In Manhattan, this would be the place to turn to. Other communities furnish a similar service.

In addition, there is a movement in the making that may be of immeasurable help to a great many aged. It has not heretofore been available but may be in action by the time this book appears in print. It is the institution of conservatorship, which means protection of "the infirm, incapacitated and confused" aged. The institution of guardianship has been in existence for a good many years, but guardianship ends when the assets of the protected person are exhausted—although it is actually then that the oldster most needs someone to look after him. The conservatorship intends to do just that. The Community Service Society of New York launched this movement, and, after long debates, the New York State Legislature enacted the proposal into law. Unfortunately, the machinery for implementing it has not yet been completed. It is a very much needed measure designed for those who have no family and cannot manage their affairs themselves. Parallel federal measures will be placed before Congress in the near future. In case a conservator is needed, the social-service department of any hospital or nursing home will know what steps to take to secure one.

ORGANIZATIONS

Organizations for social and educational purposes are listed elsewhere in this section. Others have the aim of improving the lot of the aged in general, and still others deal with individual counseling and consultation in the process of reorientation after retirement. The latter are usually connected with mental-hygiene clinics and social-service agencies.

Other organizations are centered around the community of interests among their members: unions maintain branches for their retired members, as do associations of former government employees, professionals, etc. Any retired worker can find out from his union's headquarters where the nearest branch for senior members of his organization is located, and where he can participate in social events and also play a part in the good fight for improvement of retirees' lives.

There are also national organizations with chapters in most states for aged people who are interested in public service and who wish to help in the representation of the aged in relation to the general public and to their legislators. The largest and probably the most active ones are:

The American Association of Retired Persons
1909 K Street, N.W.
Washington, D.C., 20006

The Gray Panthers
Tabernacle Church
3700 Chestnut Street
Philadelphia, Pa. 19104

The National Council of Senior Citizens
1511 K Street
Washington, D.C. 20005

National Retired Teachers Association
701 N. Montgomery Street
Ojai, Calif. 93203

The Retired Professional Action Group
c/o Public Citizen [Ralph Nader]
PO Box 19404
Washington, D.C. 20036

There are also a number of smaller local organizations with similar aims about which one can best get information from local sources.

A special group of organizations for the retired deserves mention: the various clubs whose members are all retired executives. There are quite a number of them with chapters all over the country, such as The Old Guard, based in Summit, New Jersey; The Fossils, in Washington, D.C.; and the Retired Professional and Businessmen's Club, in Santa Barbara, California. While these clubs cater primarily to the social needs of their members, there are also a number of other organizations that furnish counseling and other services to former executives. For more detailed information and other very valuable advice to retired people, see Harold Geist's book *The Psychological Aspects of Retirement.*

RECREATION

Quite a few places exist where the aged can turn for companionship and diversion. Religious organizations of all denominations maintain day centers for their aged members and neighbors. A great many national philanthropic organizations do the same, and the large cities also provide day centers for their senior citizens. Most of these facilities also offer hot meals at nominal prices.

All in all, it should not be difficult for any aged person to locate such a place simply by asking another old person in his neighborhood. If he is too shy to do so, the Information Bureau of the Community Council of Greater New York, 225 Park Avenue, New York, N.Y. 10003; telephone: 777-5000, for instance, will supply the information desired. Every large community has such an information center. In smaller communities, the local religious organizations are the places to ask for referral.

The abundance of these places can be gathered from the fact that in 1965 there were 160 such day centers in Manhattan alone. The other boroughs had fewer, but still sufficient numbers to be located within walking distance of everyone who was interested in joining.

Quite a number of movie theaters offer aged patrons reduced admission for daytime performances during the week. The identification card issued to obtain reduced fares on public-transportation facilities serves the same purpose for theater admissions. Museums are not overcrowded during the week.

SOCIAL SERVICES

It is unlikely that any aged person will want to make contact with a social agency independently. In case of financial need, the public welfare agency is the place to turn to; medical needs can be taken care of in a doctor's office or hospital; and legal matters should be handled through lawyers. All these branches of human affairs have contact with social-service agencies, and it would be best to make use of the agencies' counsel through them.

TRANSPORTATION

Almost universally, in larger cities, public-transportation fares are reduced for the aged during nonrush hours. On holidays and weekends, the reductions are in force all day. Any office for the aged will give you the telephone number of the agency administering reduced fares; a call there will tell you the place nearest your home where you can get an identification card. If you lose yours, a telephone call to this agency will bring you a replacement within a few days.

Difficulties in transportation may arise in smaller communities and suburbs without public transportation. Even if an old person owns a car, he or she should not drive after dark, if at all. Vision and hearing are not what they used to be in younger years. In some communities during the hours the children are in school, school buses are used to transport groups of old people to church services, doctors' offices, and shopping districts. Volunteer car pools have also been arranged for these purposes, and more are being formed.

VOLUNTEER ACTIVITIES

The interrelation between the rewards derived from doing volunteer work and the benefit to the recipient has been described in detail in Chapter 7. Therefore, I shall confine myself here to listing the places where older, especially retired, workers can find self-ful-fillment by enrolling in one of the organizations that could not function without them.

First, there are all the religious and philanthropic organizations that need people to work for them without compensation or for a token payment. Every house of worship of any denomination has a corps of people of all ages and both sexes who devote time and effort to helping others in any capacity they can. Hospitals, nursing homes, and public institutions for the mentally and physically handicapped rely heavily on the unselfish interest with which the volunteers augment the efforts of the professional staff.

The government has lately become aware of untapped manpower possibilities, not only in the interest of the recipients but also in the interest of the donors and their time and knowledge. It has established a series of organizations in which all adults, particularly retirees, can become active again and by their contributions regain their self-esteem and perhaps make a little money besides. The program itself, under the auspices of the Department of Health, Education, and Welfare, is called ACTION. Its several subgroups—none of which has an age limit, and all of which welcome the elderly—include:

The Peace Corps. works in foreign countries, and VISTA (Volunteers in Service to America), does the same kind of work within our fifty states. Foster Grandparents, which has become very popular among both parties, offers love and care to children who need both. RSVP (Retired Senior Volunteer Program) gives its services to activities within its local communities. SCORE (Service Corps for Retired Executives) consists of members who share their knowledge and experience to counsel small business owners on management problems.

Detailed information about these agencies can be obtained by writing to: ACTION, Washington, D.C. 20525.

While the lot of many aged people is not a very enviable one and while they complain with justification that they are unwanted and unloved, we see that there is a tremendous stirring among the concerned members of our population as well as the federal government, with all its state and local branches, making great efforts to improve the situation of their elders. There are more facilities for making their lives easier than even an informed and curious citizen would ever imagine. More and better publicity would do a world of good, especially if it came from the aged themselves. Let me be among the avant-garde.

Appendix B

SOURCES USED IN PREPARING THIS STUDY AND OTHER RECOMMENDED WRITINGS

Recommended Reading

Berry, Frank B., ed. "Introduction to Old Age," *Bulletin of the New York Academy of Medicine*, vol. 47, no. 11, November 1971.

"Conservatorship," *Bulletin of the Community Service Society of New York*, vol. 721, January 1973.

Cummings, Elaine, and Henry, William E. *Growing Old: The Process of Disengagement*. New York: Basic Books, 1961.

Curtin, Sharon R. *Nobody Ever Died of Old Age*. Boston: Atlantic Monthly Press, 1973.

De Beauvoir, Simone. *The Coming of Age: The Study of the Aging Process*. New York: Putnam, 1972. Paperback edition: paperback Library, 1973.

Dependencies of Old People, The. Occasional Papers in Gerontology, no. 6. Ann Arbor: Institute of Gerontology, University of Michigan and Wayne State University, 1969.

Directory of Senior Citizens. Washington, D.C.: Superintendent of Documents, U.S. Government Printing Office.

Directory of Services for the Aging in New York State. Albany, N.Y.: New York State (revised annually).

Education for Aging. Albany, N.Y.: University of the State of New York.

Farnsworth, Dana L. "Preparing for Retirement," *Psychiatric Annals—Geriatrics*, Part II, vol. 2, no. 11, November 1972.

Field, Minna. *The Aged, the Family, and the Community*. New York: Columbia University Press, 1972.

Freud, Sigmund. *Three Essays on the Theory of Sexuality*. New York: Basic Books, 1962. Paperback edition: Avon, 1971.

Fuchs, Lawrence H. *Family Matters*. New York: Random House, 1972.

Geist, Harold. *The Psychological Aspects of Retirement*. Springfield, Ill.: C. C. Thomas, 1968.

Geist, Harold. *The Psychological Aspects of the Aging Process: With Sociological Implications*. St. Louis: Warren H. Green, 1969.

Hendin, David. *Death as a Fact of Life*. New York: Norton, 1973. Paperback edition: Warner Paperback Library, 1974.

Housing. Washington, D.C.: U.S. Department of Housing and Urban Development.

Kaufman, M. Ralph. "Old Age and Aging: The Psychoanalytic View," *American Journal of Orthopsychiatry*, vol. 10, no. 1, January 1940.

Kavaler, Florence, *et al*. "Proprietary Nursing Homes in New York City," *Bulletin of the New York Academy of Medicine* (New York), vol. 49, no. 9, September 1973.

Knopf, Olga. "Aging," *Mount Sinai Journal of Medicine* (New York), vol. 39, no. 4, July–August, 1972.

Kubie, Susan H., and Landau, Gertrude. *Group Work with the Aged*. New York: International Universities Press, 1969.

Lehman, Virginia. *You, the Law, and Retirement*. Washington, D.C.: Social and Rehabilitation Service, Administration on Aging, U.S. Department of Health, Education, and Welfare, 1972.

Living in a Multigeneration Family. Occasional Papers in Gerontology, no. 3. Ann Arbor: Institute of Gerontology, University of Michigan and Wayne State University, 1969.

Martin, Peter A. *Leisure and Mental Health: A Psychiatric Viewpoint*. Washington, D.C.: Committee on Leisure Time and Its Uses, American Psychiatric Association, 1967.

"Meeting the Problems of Older People, the 1973 Health Conference," *Bulletin of the New York Academy of Medicine* (New York), vol. 49, no. 12, December 1973.

Mitchell, William L. *Preparation for Retirement: A New Guide to Program Development for Business and Industry.* Washington, D.C.: American Association of Retired Persons, 1969.

Nader, Ralph, and Blackwell, Kate. *You and Your Pension.* New York: Grossman, 1973.

Nursing Home Care. Washington, D.C.: Social and Rehabilitation Service, Administration on Aging, U.S. Department of Health, Education, and Welfare, 1973.

Poe, William D. *The Old Person in the House.* New York: Scribner's, 1969.

Recreation for the Elderly. Albany: University of the State of New York (revised annually).

Regan, John J. "Protective Services for the Elderly: Commitment, Guardianship and Alternatives," *William and Mary Law Review,* vol. 13, no. 3, Spring 1972.

Resources for the Aging: An Action Handbook. Washington, D.C.: Office of Economic Opportunity,

Retirement Planning: A "How To" Guide for Organizing and Conducting Group Programs. New York: Office for the Aging, Office of the Mayor, 1973.

Rome, Howard P. "Introductory Remarks," *Psychiatric Annals—Geriatrics,* Part I, vol. 2, no. 10, October 1972.

Rubin, Isadore. *Sexual Life after Sixty.* New York: Basic Books, 1965.

Sherman, Susan R. "Satisfaction and Retirement Housing," *Aging and Human Development,* vol. 3, no. 4, November 1972.

Shock, Nathan W. *Trends in Gerontology.* Second edition. San Francisco; Stanford University Press, 1957.

Simmons, Leo W. *The Role of the Aged in Primitive Society,* New Haven: Yale University Press, 1945; reprinted 1970 by Shoe String Press, Hamden, Connecticut.

Simon, Alexander, and Epstein, Leon J., eds. *Aging in Modern Society.* Report no. 23. New York: American Psychiatric Association, 1967–68.

Social Security: The First Thirty-Five Years. Occasional Papers in

Gerontology, no. 7. Ann Arbor: Institute of Gerontology, University of Michigan and Wayne State University, 1970.

Tibbitts, Clark, ed. *Handbook of Social Gerontology: Societal Aspects of Aging.* Chicago: University of Chicago Press, 1960.

Townsend, Claire, project director. *Old Age, The Last Segregation: The Report on Nursing Homes* (Ralph Nader's Study Group Reports). New York: Grossman, 1971.

Trends in Early Retirement. Occasional Papers in Gerontology, no. 4. Ann Arbor: Institute of Gerontology, University of Michigan and Wayne State University, 1969.

White House Conference on Aging. *Toward a National Policy on Aging.* 2 vols. Washington, D.C.: U.S. Government Printing Office, 1971–73.

Williams, T. F., *et al.* "Appropriate Placement of the Chronically Ill and Aged," *Journal of the American Medical Association,* vol. 226, no. 11, December 1973.

Zimring, Joseph G. "The Right to Die with Dignity," *New York State Journal of Medicine,* Vol. 73, no. 13, July 1, 1973.

Zinberg, Norman E., and Kaufman, Irving, eds., *Normal Psychology of the Aging Process.* New York: International Universities Press, 1963.

Periodicals

Aging (monthly). Administration on Aging, U.S. Department of Health, Education, and Welfare, U.S. Government Printing Office, Washington, D.C. 20402

Cameo Newsletter. New York State, Office for the Aging, 112 State Street, Albany, N.Y. 12201

Current Literature on Aging (quarterly). National Council on the Aging, 1828 L Street, N.W. Washington, D.C. 20036

Directory of Services for the Aging in New York State (annual). New York State, 112 State Street, Albany, N.Y. 12201

Gerontologist, The (bimonthly). The Gerontological Society, 1 Dupont Circle, Washington, D.C. 20036

International Journal of Aging and Human Development (quarterly). Baywood Publishing Corp., 43 Central Drive, Farmingdale, N.Y. 11735

Journal of the American Geriatrics Society (monthly). 10 Columbus Circle, New York, N.Y. 10019

Modern Maturity (every second month). American Association of Retired Persons, 215 Long Beach Boulevard, Long Beach, Calif. 90801 accidents, home, avoidance of, 118

ACE, 197

ACTION, 4, 197, 216, 217

activity: importance of, 53; indoor, 70-71; reduction in, 23; outdoor, 70. *See also* athletics; inactivity

age-consciousness, 29-30

aged persons. *See* senior citizens

aging: awareness of, 189; concept of, 13-14; denial of, 41-42, 189-190; effect on children, 142-43; emotional responses to, 21-27; functional changes in, 18-19; manifestation of, 15; personality and, 24-26; signs of, camouflage of, 31-32; society and, 29. *See also* healthy aging

American Association of Retired Persons, 64, 204

anxiety related to senior citizens, 22. *See also* stress

apathy, 82-83

appearance, 11; maintenance of, 122-23

athletics, compromises in, 29, 69-70

balance, sense of, impairment of, 17

Bellin, Lowell E., 167

Blenkner, Margaret, 44

cancer. *See* malignancy

care of aged: "coordinated home-care program," 158-59; Foster Home Care, 159; organizations concerned with, 89-91; sheltered workshop, 91-92; visiting nurse, 128. *See also* day centers; geriatric centers; nursing homes

cataract, treatment of, 119

children: financial aid from, 139-140; living with, 136-37, 143-146; relations between parents and, 140-43, 146-47. *See also* relationships, family

cleanliness. *See* hygiene

comfort, physical, need for, 35-36